THE POWER OF
ENERGY HEALING

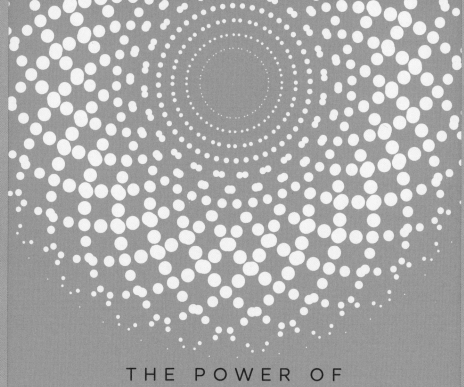

THE POWER OF
ENERGY HEALING

SIMPLE PRACTICES TO PROMOTE WELLBEING

VICTOR ARCHULETA

FAIR WINDS

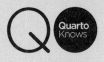

Inspiring | Educating | Creating | Entertaining

Brimming with creative inspiration, how-to projects, and useful information to enrich your everyday life, Quarto Knows is a favorite destination for those pursuing their interests and passions. Visit our site and dig deeper with our books into your area of interest: Quarto Creates, Quarto Cooks, Quarto Homes, Quarto Lives, Quarto Drives, Quarto Explores, Quarto Gifts, or Quarto Kids.

First published in 2021 by Fair Winds Press, an imprint of The Quarto Group. 100 Cummings Center, Suite 265-D, Beverly, MA 01915, USA. T (978) 282-9590 F (978) 283-2742

Fair Winds Press titles are also available at discount for retail, wholesale, promotional, and bulk purchase. For details, contact the Special Sales Manager by email at specialsales@quarto. com or by mail at The Quarto Group, Attn: Special Sales Manager, 100 Cummings Center, Suite 265-D, Beverly, MA 01915, USA.

24 23 22 21 20 1 2 3 4 5

ISBN: 978-1-58923-995-1

Digital edition published in 2021

QUAR.340579

Conceived, edited, and designed by Quarto Publishing plc. 6 Blundell Street, London N7 9BH

Senior Commissioning Editor: Eszter Karpati
Editor: Caroline West
Project Editor: Anna Galkina
Art Director: Gemma Wilson
Designer: Karin Skånberg
Illustrator: Dmytro Yurchenko (except illustrations credited on page 128)
Junior Designer: India Minter
Publisher: Samantha Warrington

Printed in Singapore

The information in this book is for educational purposes only. It is not intended to replace the advice of a physician or medical practitioner. Please see your health-care provider before beginning any new health program.

Contents

About This Book 6

Introduction 10

CHAPTER 1
BASIC PRINCIPLES OF
ENERGY HEALING 12

Understanding Energy Healing 14

Energetic Flow and How
It is Used for Healing 16

Energy Concepts 18

Energy Fields and Forces 20

Meditations and Visualizations
to Focus and Direct
Energy Healing 24

CHAPTER 2
AILMENTS DIRECTORY 26

Homeostasis: Striving Toward
a Same-state Condition 28

The Ailments 30

Physiological Ailments 32

Psychological Ailments 40

Mechanical Ailments 44

CHAPTER 3
THE ENERGY HEALING ARTS 46

Movement Therapies 48

Energy Flow Therapies 62

Bioenergetic Therapies 68

Meditation Energy Therapies 82

Directed Energy Therapies 88

CHAPTER 4
HEALING EXERCISES 92

1 Energization Exercises 94

2 Finger Qigong Exercises 104

3 The Five Tibetan Rites Exercise 108

4 Deep Relaxation and Pressure
Point Technique Exercises 114

Glossary 120

Index 126

Further resources 128

Acknowledgments 128

Illustration credits 128

About This Book

This book takes you through some background information on energy healing in Chapter 1, including its key principles. In Chapter 2, you will learn about which energy healing modalities and exercises can be used to address a variety of issues and ailments. Chapter 3 describes these modalities in more depth, and you can follow step-by-step guides to healing exercises in Chapter 4. Finally, a Glossary at the back of the book provides explanations of any terms you may be unsure about.

CHAPTER 1
BASIC PRINCIPLES OF ENERGY HEALING
pages 12–25
Describes the basic principles of energy, and covers how these principles affect our mind, body, and spirit, and why they are relevant to energy as medicine.

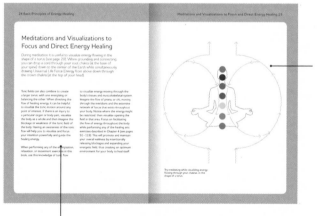

Helpful illustrations bring the energy healing principles to life.

Dive into the ideas and history behind energy healing, so you can give yourself a theoretical foundation on which to build your healing practice.

CHAPTER 2
AILMENTS DIRECTORY
pages 26–45

Contains an Ailments Directory that describes common types of disease, (divided into broad categories of ailments), along with suggestions for energy exercises from Chapter 4 to address the issue or concern.

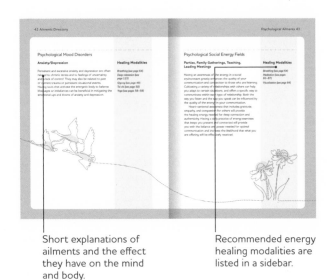

Short explanations of ailments and the effect they have on the mind and body.

Recommended energy healing modalities are listed in a sidebar.

CHAPTER 3
THE ENERGY HEALING ARTS
pages 46–91

Describes different types of energy healing modalities and therapies, providing information on the level of difficulty, materials required, and any limitations to performing them.

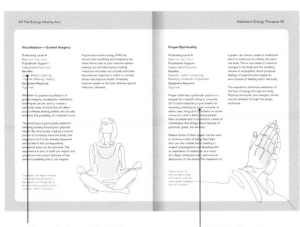

Short bulleted lists give a quick overview of each therapy or practice, making it simple to choose the right one for your need.

An introduction to each modality follows, giving more detail and background information.

CHAPTER 4
HEALING EXERCISES
pages 92-119
Provides information on specific healing arts exercises,
with step-by-step instructions of how to perform them
so you can achieve a particular goal in energy healing.

Brief introduction to each exercise, with
background information and history.

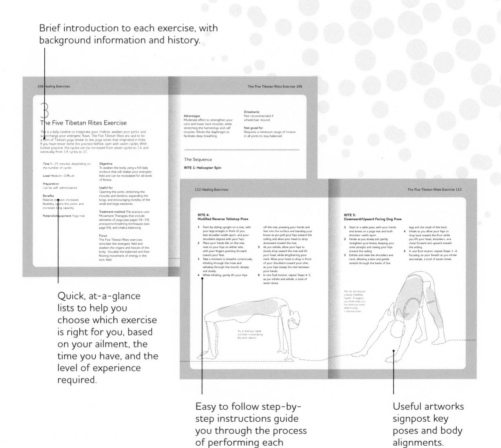

Quick, at-a-glance
lists to help you
choose which exercise
is right for you, based
on your ailment, the
time you have, and the
level of experience
required.

Easy to follow step-by-
step instructions guide
you through the process
of performing each
healing exercise.

Useful artworks
signpost key
poses and body
alignments.

GLOSSARY
pages 120–125
A Glossary at the back of the book provides a helpful reference of terms that can be found throughout each chapter.

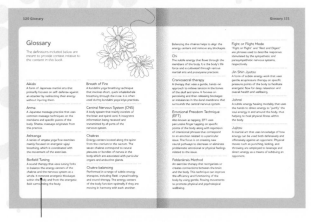

If you come across an unfamiliar word, you can find it easily in this alphabetical glossary.

Disclaimer

This book is not intended as a means of diagnosing illness or disease, nor is it meant to prescribe treatments for curing illness or disease. Wherever the words "heal" or "healing" appear, it is intended that the protocols themselves do not "heal," but rather facilitate the body's own ability to heal itself.

While many of these protocols may be useful, it is important to note that, in general, they are not supported by scientific research or evidence-based studies. Any physical or mental health challenges you may be experiencing should be addressed by a qualified physician and/or psychotherapist.

Introduction

Energy healing primarily exists in a domain outside of traditional allopathic or Western medicine. The intention of this book is to familiarize readers with energy healing and to encourage them to experiment with energy-healing practices. It does not attempt to provide "scientific proof" to support the therapies nor reference any research studies that aim to do so.

Exploring energy as medicine is a journey into embracing a more right-brained approach. If you're mostly analytical and methodical in your thinking, you're said to be left-brained. If you tend to be more creative or artistic, you're thought to be right-brained. This approach does not need to understand, know, believe, or prove an experience, but instead opts to trust in and allow an experience as it unfolds. Most of these energy-healing phenomena exist in fields of energy that cannot easily be measured by modern science. If we acknowledge that because of technical limitations in measuring subtle energy forces, proving the efficacy of energy healing is not possible, then we are able to focus on using intuition and intention to have an experience of energy and observe what occurs.

The practice of using energy to improve the wellbeing of others has been around for millennia. In biblical times, energy was directed from one person to another by healers who performed a "laying on of hands" to heal illness and disease. Today, modern clergy continue to bestow blessings on the faithful by holding the palms of their hands toward the congregation during a service.

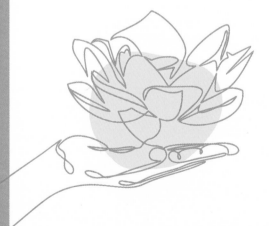

Historically, indigenous tribes around the world have used energy healing medicine, reciting prayers and blessings, as well as using herbs and plants, in sacred ceremonies. The yogis of India, along with the Hindu and Buddhist monks of Asia, developed meditation practices and types of martial arts that facilitated the flow of the Universal Life Force Energy (also known as prana or chi/qi) for healing purposes. More recently, kings and sorcerers of medieval Europe, as well as early American witches, were known to use incantations and to curse or cast spells on their enemies.

Ancient energy healing and wellness processes have evolved into a variety of yoga and meditation practices and subtle energy medicine modalities such as *Reiki* (see page 89), *Reflexology* (see page 72), *Craniosacral Therapy* (see page 72), *Polarity Therapy* (see page 74), *Jin Shin Jyutsu* (see page 73), and *Johrei* (see page 90). Using both subtle energy practices and physical exercise, we can intentionally affect the body's energetic fields for healing purposes. Having an awareness of what energy is and how it works, we can then seek out and access the power of energy healing to address specific issues and so promote health and wellbeing.

Benefits of Energy Healing

Various conditions can be helped by utilizing some of the energy healing therapies described in this book. Some common conditions that can benefit from energy healing include:

- Physical pain and discomfort caused by injuries, ailments, and diseases.
- Tension and stress due to the anxiety and uncertainty of living in the modern world.
- Headaches and neck, shoulder, and back pain caused by a lack of exercise and a sedentary lifestyle (which have become commonplace in today's world).
- Emotional imbalances that occur as a result of daily interactions with others who are also experiencing extraordinary challenges.

These conditions may manifest in a variety of physiological, psychological, and mechanical ailments. By following the step-by-step exercises presented in this book you can influence existing fields to address specific ailments and use the power of energy healing to optimize your overall wellness and help maintain a healthy lifestyle.

CHAPTER 1
BASIC PRINCIPLES OF ENERGY HEALING

When you first encounter energy healing, it can seem like a mysterious and esoteric practice that involves an element of magical thinking, or rituals of prayer and chanting, to spontaneously heal an injury or disease. There are no pills to take or procedures to follow, so how can energy actually heal?

Understanding Energy Healing

To better understand energy healing, it is useful to look at some of the key principles and concepts involved. A basic understanding of what energy is, how it is used, what it looks like, and how it is experienced can provide a foundation for harnessing energy and using it to heal ourselves. The power of energy healing is available to anyone who is willing to step into the realm of mystery and magic, attempt to answer these questions, and experience it for themselves.

What is Energy?

In its simplest terms, energy can be defined as any measurable force that originates from one object and is transferred to another.

Energy exists in many forms, including electrical, magnetic, thermal, and physical forces. Science has been able to quantify and measure many different types of energy. This has resulted in the development of many amazing and magical technologies in modern life. Although we may not understand the specifics of how a cell phone works, for example, we know that the technology is scientifically sound. However, if someone from the early 20th century were to encounter one, it would seem like a kind of magical, if not heretical, device that might be associated with some type of dark force.

Science offers proof of how and why things are the way they are. Regardless of the existence of anecdotal or empirical

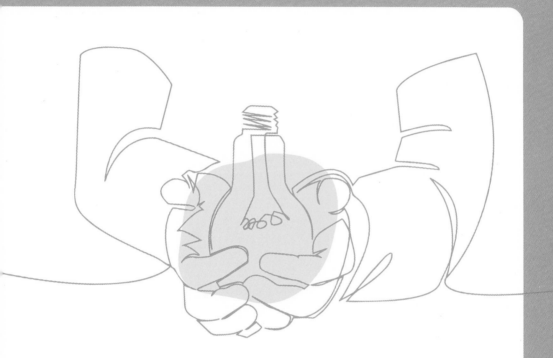

evidence, if science is unable to measure or quantify the energetic effects of a specific healing practice, it will often be assumed that the practice is not to be relied upon. These phenomena are regarded as magical or mysterious until they are studied and understood by science.

Being aware of this situation gives us an opportunity to explore the effectiveness of energy-healing practices by trying them out for ourselves in the absence of any scientific proof. Although scientists may one day develop ways to prove the efficacy of energy healing, perhaps we can still derive benefit from the practice without actual proof of how or why it works. The "proof is in the pudding," and if the expected result is achieved, then empirical evidence is just as good as scientific proof.

Energetic Flow and How It is Used for Healing

One of the many characteristics of some types of energy is that it can only be measured by potential differences between two points. Differences in potential energy can be measured between a source (in the case of energy healing, this is the practitioner) and a target (the client/patient), and these measurements can be used to demonstrate that there is an actual flow of energy between the two points. If the strength and direction of the flow can be determined, it is easier to understand the effect that the energy from a source is having on the target.

There are many systems in the body that want to keep things moving. Some include the flow of energy through the chakra vortexes or the energy lines of meridians. Other systems operate on a more physical level. The circulation of blood and lymphatic fluids, the movement of air in the respiratory system, the transmission of electrical nerve impulses in the nervous system, the digestion of food in the gastrointestinal system, and the motion in the musculoskeletal system all perform best when they are flowing smoothly. So it is apparent that optimal health is achieved when there is flow in all bodily systems.

Conversely, blocked or impeded flow is a recipe for possible injury, and creates an environment for disease or dysfunction.

When an energy healer is working on a client, it may seem as if some type of intervention is occurring. But what is the state of this energetic flow? How and where is the energy moving? It may be that the practitioner is directing energy toward the client for a particular reason. Alternatively, the practitioner may be gleaning information by sensing or feeling energy from the client to determine how or where to apply energy in return.

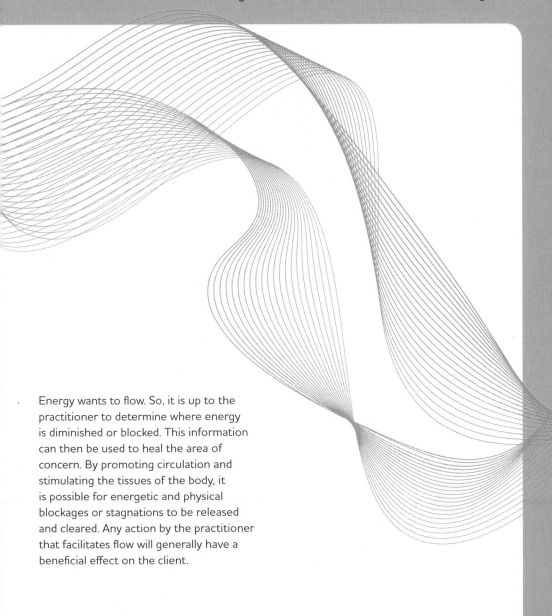

Energy wants to flow. So, it is up to the practitioner to determine where energy is diminished or blocked. This information can then be used to heal the area of concern. By promoting circulation and stimulating the tissues of the body, it is possible for energetic and physical blockages or stagnations to be released and cleared. Any action by the practitioner that facilitates flow will generally have a beneficial effect on the client.

Energy Concepts

Learning about some of the key concepts behind energy can help you understand its different characteristics, aspects, and properties. These concepts are explained over the next few pages and include an understanding of the physical receptors of stimuli from our environment and an awareness of energetic fields and their shape. An awareness of these concepts will provide a context for the ideas explored in *Chapter 4 Healing Exercises* (see pages 92–119).

Energy and the Five Senses

The five senses all provide inputs to our bodies that help us perceive our environment. Energy is the primary conveyor of stimuli, which we are able to perceive using our senses. The extent to which we are able to perceive our environment is proportional to the variety of experiences we can have. The more keenly aware we are of our senses, the richer our experience will be.

Color, sound, smell, taste, and touch, and whole body senses, all provide information to help us experience and interact with the world around us. We are able to use this information to harness the specific types of energy needed for healing.

Sight may be perceived as frequencies of light that are either reflected off surfaces or emitted by a light source. Although these are similar, the body can have a different energetic response, depending on the source. For example, walking into a room lit only by red lights evokes a different response than walking into a room with four red walls. One can be grounding and calming, while the other can be energizing and anxiety-provoking. It is worth exploring the use of various color frequencies as a non-invasive form of energy healing medicine to address energetic imbalances, physical injuries, and certain diseases and ailments.

Sound In a similar way to sight, the vibration of sound can have a powerful effect on the body, depending on how it is applied. A single-tone sound frequency can help reset the individual chakra energy centers. Or when different tones are combined, sound can be experienced as harmonious, soothing, and pleasing or discordant, agitating, and upsetting. Sound can also be either energizing or relaxing. Because the body is mostly composed of water, some frequencies actually penetrate through the skin and have a physical effect as well. The percussive vibration of sound literally shakes and opens up the connective tissue between the organs of the body. This opening can increase circulation within the tissues and energetically clear pathways of all sorts of things to promote unobstructed flow. Sound and vibration can be used to alter or reset an unbalanced system and promote healing.

Smell and taste are completely intertwined. Put simply, these senses work as a result of chemical molecules attaching to receptors that perceive smell and taste. These receptors include sweet, sour, salty, bitter, or a combination of these. The senses are often tied to specific memories and can be used to process past traumas or upsetting events.

Touch Receptors just below the surface of the skin respond to temperature, pressure, texture, and pain. Much of the information that is received by touch receptors is used unconsciously. Your body knows exactly how to interact with its environment in a smooth, seamless way. Touch can provide extraordinary energetic experiences. It is tied to deep feelings of intimacy, connection, and nurturing. The flow of energy through the body can be influenced by external stimuli that are perceived through receptors in the skin.

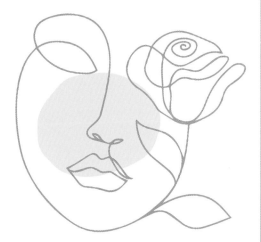

Essential oils

Working on a number of the senses, particularly smell and touch, the molecules of essential oils are easily absorbed through the skin and through the nose, and have immediate and specific effects on mood, emotions, and physical wellbeing. Essential oils can be used to provide pain relief, and they may have a calming or energizing effect, depending on the situation being addressed. They can also be used to help facilitate the healing of injuries and ailments, and even cause a shift in the energetic field of the body.

Energy Fields and Forces

The idea of an energy transmitter and a receiver is fairly well understood and has been experienced by many people. It is also easy to accept that a signal is being sent and received. These signals consist of modulated energy waveforms transmitted through some type of medium. The medium can be the atmosphere, which is needed for the transmission of signals for AM/FM radio, television, cell phones, and Wi-Fi, or it can be a physical medium such as 20th-century telephone lines used for a landline call.

If we take the concept of transmitting and receiving energy a step beyond technological inventions like Wi-Fi, we can imagine our physical bodies as very complex receivers (sensory receptors) and transmitters (bioelectric fields) of many different types of energy waveforms. These waveforms typically have the characteristics of frequency and amplitude, which can otherwise be understood as pulse and strength. This type of energy can also be measured in the bioelectric field of the body.

Whether it is our hearts generating a signal in the form of an electrocardiogram (EKG), our brains generating an electroencephalogram (EEG), or our life energy moving along the meridians of our bodies, energy is constantly being generated and transferred. Hence, our bodies consist of a system of intricately designed antennae and transmitters that detect and transfer information within and outside the body. We sense things through the movement of energy, which affects how we perceive ourselves and the world around us.

What is a Torus?

An important characteristic of energy is the concept of flow. If the energy-transfer system is not flowing, then the energy transmission will be ineffective and the system will not function. When energy moves freely, it flows in a particular direction and has a specific shape called a torus. The toric flow of energy occurs at all levels of physical existence. Matter in any form or size emits an electromagnetic

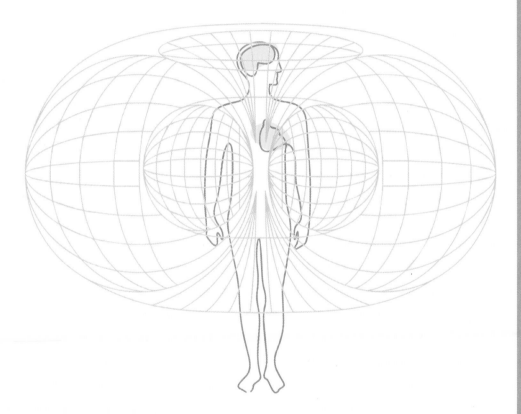

The rhythmic electromagentic
field generated by the heart is
the largest of any organ.

field in the shape of a torus. This is true for individual atoms, molecules, cells, tissues, organs, and bodies, as well as planets, solar systems, and even galaxies. A toric field looks like the cross section of an apple that has been cut in half vertically through the stem. A more 3-D toric representation is visible when the Earth's magnetic field is ionized and creates the amazing light shows of the aurora borealis and the aurora australis. The toric field of the Earth allows energy to flow down from the "north" pole, through the center of the torus, out the "south" pole, and then

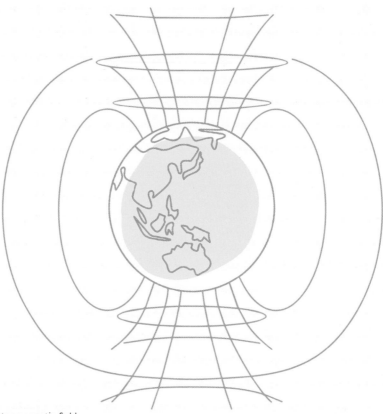

The electromagentic field generated by the Earth can be seen in the Northern Hemisphere as the Aurora Borealis.

to circle up around the planet and back to the "north" pole in a continuous motion. The flow occurs in the opposite direction as well. Another way to visualize a toric field is to imagine energy flowing in spirals in opposite directions around the surface of a donut. It is important to understand this type of energy flow while performing energy healing.

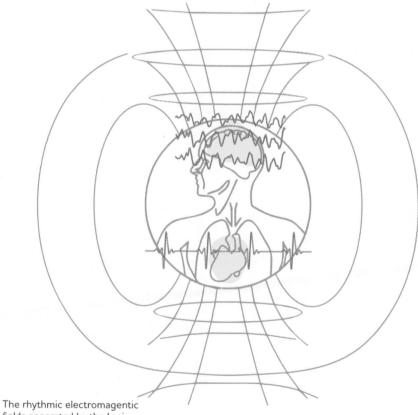

The rhythmic electromagentic fields generated by the brain and the heart are strong enough to be measured.

Meditations and Visualizations to Focus and Direct Energy Healing

During meditation it is useful to visualize energy flowing in the shape of a torus (see page 20). When grounding and connecting, you can drop a cord through your root chakra (at the base of your spine) down to the center of the Earth while simultaneously drawing Universal Life Force Energy from above down through the crown chakra (at the top of your head).

Toric fields can also combine to create a larger torus, with one energizing or balancing the other. When directing the flow of healing energy, it can be helpful to visualize the toric motion around any point of interest. If there is an injury to a particular organ or body part, visualize the body as a whole and then imagine the blockage or weakness of the toric field of the body. Having an awareness of the toric flow will help you to visualize and focus your intention powerfully and guide the healing energy.

When performing any of the energization, relaxation, or movement exercises in this book, use this knowledge of toric flow to visualize energy moving through the body's tissues and musculoskeletal system. Imagine the flow of prana, or chi, moving through the meridians and the extensive network of fascia that exists throughout your body. Notice where the energy might be restricted, then visualize opening the field in that area. Focus on facilitating the flow of energy throughout the body while performing any of the healing arts exercises described in Chapter 4 (see pages 92–119). This will promote and maintain your overall wellness by intentionally releasing blockages and expanding your energetic field, thus creating an optimum environment for your body to heal itself.

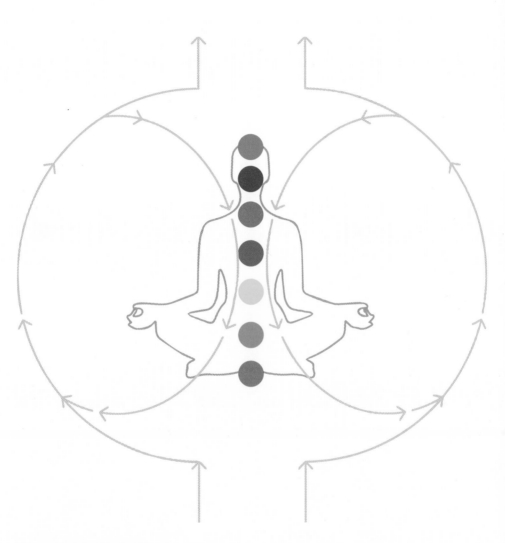

Try meditating while visualizing energy flowing through your chakras, in the shape of a torus.

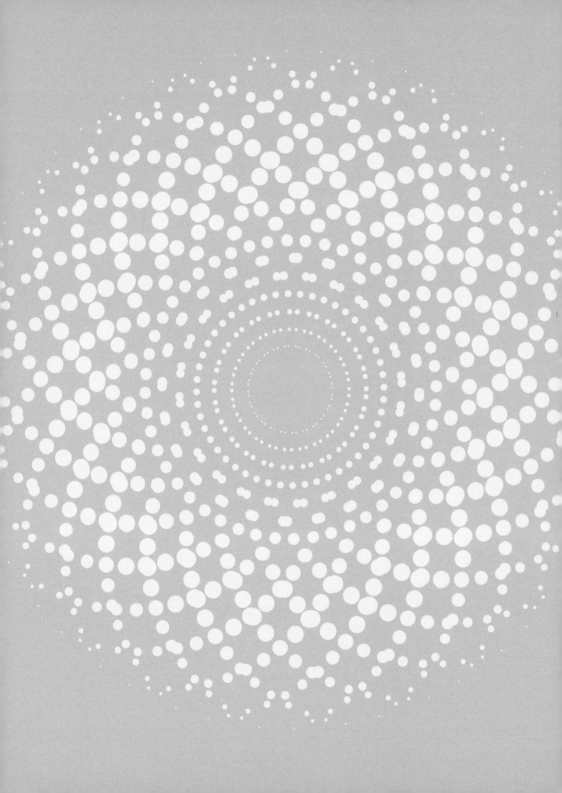

CHAPTER 2
AILMENTS DIRECTORY

In this chapter you will find an overview of common physiological, psychological, and mechanical ailments, with suggestions for energy healing modalities that can alleviate stress, pain, and heal both body and mind.

HOMEOSTASIS: Striving Toward a Same-state Condition

The human body is composed of a variety of intricately balanced, distinct, and interdependent systems. These systems rely upon a finely orchestrated network of communications for optimal functioning. Both internal and external forces can upset the balance of the body's systems. However, in an effort to maintain homeostasis, ongoing adjustments to the systems naturally occur to return them to a balanced state.

When the body is unbalanced due to poor diet, a sedentary lifestyle, smoking, medicating with drugs or alcohol, or situational stress, it will attempt to optimize the functioning of the various systems to provide the best possible outcome in a given situation.

The body will try to achieve homeostasis in a variety of ways. The release of hormones and neurotranmitters can be used to affect the balance of electrolytes across cell membranes and adjust blood pressure to balance the system. These hormonal adjustments may also affect the glucose levels in the body in an attempt to bring the system back to a balanced state. With acute or one-off disruptions, the body can be highly effective in restoring balance. However, when the disruption to a system is chronic or unrelenting, the body will attempt to signal that something is wrong so that the disruption can be minimized or eliminated. These signals may manifest as feelings of discomfort and even pain at or near the site of disruption.

Persistant signals that present as chronic pain and discomfort can easily cause anxiety or depression over time. This may lead to the use of pharmaceutical medications to reduce pain and relieve depression or anxiety, thus addressing the symptoms of the problem rather than resolving the underlying condition. This can then increase the overall disruption of the system. If an issue is left unaddressed, the body will find more ways to get your attention by increasing the levels

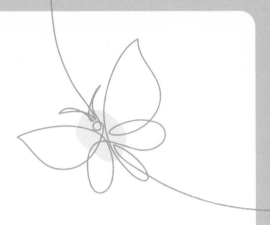

of physical pain and compromising the functioning of the affected systems, and disease may eventually be the result.

Ailments and diseases that are caused by unbalanced conditions may manifest in a variety of physiological, psychological, and mechanical systems. The amount of energy needed to maintain homeostasis is increased in proportion to the level of imbalance that is present. Any intervention that promotes or facilitates balance, and the proper flow of the body's systems, will decrease the energetic demand on the body and free the energy for maintaining overall wellness. Having an awareness of these imbalances may provide a frame of reference to visualize and experience the flow of energy within the body and enable you to interpret when systems are in balance or out of balance, or blocked.

Fortunately, there are a number of energy-centered wellness modalities that can help develop this awareness, facilitating the body's ability to achieve homeostasis and so alleviating the pain and discomfort that results from ailments and disease. Whether it's meditation, movement medicine, therapeutic bodywork, or mindful nutrition and exercise, intentionally following a personal practice based on energy healing can help the body achieve homeostasis. Homeostasis creates an optimal environment that facilitates the body's innate ability to work around blockages, efficiently repair injured tissues, and maintain the healthy functioning and energetic flow of the various systems. This is necessary if you are to achieve a balanced, peaceful lifestyle filled with wellbeing and optimism.

The Ailments

A variety of ailments may have their origins in disruptions in, or external perturbations of, the energy fields of the body. For example, nausea or discomfort in the pit of the stomach or chronic lower back pain can transform into an ulcer or a herniated disc, respectively. If we are not intuitively aware or not conscious of how our thoughts affect our health, we may unintentionally create harmful thought patterns. Thinking or saying phrases such as "My stomach is killing me" or "So and so is a pain in my side" may produce thought patterns that energetically create an environment which may actually cause disease.

Being aware of our thoughts and belief systems can affect the health of our physical, emotional, and energetic bodies. Through the proactive use of energy-healing practices, the pain and discomfort caused by many ailments can be mitigated, or even eliminated, and the body is then able to heal itself. This Ailment Directory is your guide to understanding how the power of the energy healing arts can be accessed through the practice of energetic exercises.

Physiological Ailments

Physiological ailments, disorders, and diseases can manifest in many ways. The more obvious include habits or behaviors that directly disrupt the balance of various body systems. Poor diet, smoking, alcohol or drug abuse, and lack of exercise can all challenge the body's ability to repair damaged tissues or remove toxins. The ailments described here result in varying degrees of disruption. These can be mitigated by implementing energetic interventions to slow or eliminate the damage being done and encourage the repair and healing of the affected systems.

Cardiovascular Ailments

Heart Disease, Stroke, Chronic Obstructive Pulmonary Disease (COPD)

There are many causes of cardiovascular ailments, including smoking, high cholesterol, chronic stress, and viral diseases. Lifestyle choices that include a balanced diet, proper nutrition, physical exercise, yoga, and meditation can help decrease stress and minimize cardiovascular issues, as well as contribute to your overall health and wellness.

Having a wellness practice that includes conscious eating, a variety of stress-reducing, energy-balancing practices, and gentle body movement provides an environment for healing and may contribute to your overall cardiovascular health.

Healing Modalities

Breathing (see page 64)
Qigong (see page 49)
Tai chi (see page 50)
Yoga (see pages 58–59)

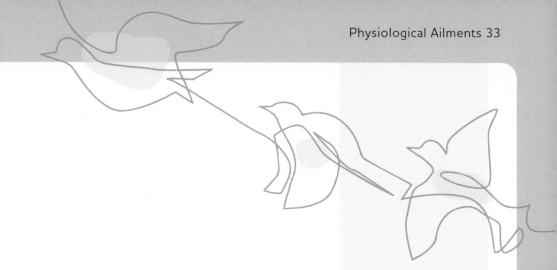

Autoimmune/Inflammatory Disorders

Rheumatoid Arthritis, Lupus, Celiac Disease, Psoriasis, Type 1 Diabetes

Rheumatoid arthritis and lupus are two chronic inflammatory autoimmune disorders that result in painful stiffness of the wrists and fingers and decreased joint mobility, and, in the case of lupus, fatigue and fever. Other autoimmune diseases, such as celiac disease, psoriasis, and type-1 diabetes, compromise the normal functioning of the gastrointestinal system and organs of the body. The effects of autoimmune disease can be debilitating and challenging, and developing practices that provide relief of any kind are welcome and can be of great benefit.

Practices that focus our intention on the present moment, even if physically painful, can provide a sense of control and relief. Instead of succumbing to the suffering associated with physical pain, it is possible to be with the pain in a way that allows you to experience it as an observer, removed from the physical feeling itself. Having a daily practice of energy-balancing techniques that promotes a calm and peaceful demeanor may help dissipate the agitation caused by chronic pain, anxiety, and discomfort.

Healing Modalities

Breathing (see page 64)

Deep relaxation (see page 115)

Meditation (see pages 82–87)

Visualization (see page 84)

Gastrointestinal Ailments

Crohn's Disease and Irritable Bowel Syndrome (IBS), Leaky Gut Syndrome

The gastrointestinal system is the first point of entry for the breakdown and absorption of all nutrients needed by the body and is the final step in the elimination of toxins, waste, and the end-products of metabolism. Poor diet and nutrition, and unmanaged stress and anxiety, can lead to gastrointestinal ailments that make it difficult to maintain a healthy lifestyle. Consuming fresh, unprocessed, nutrient-dense foods can provide the energy and nutrition needed to heal the issues that contribute to GI ailments.

A wellness practice that includes conscious eating, gentle body movement, and a diet of healthy, unprocessed foods can improve the function of the entire gastrointestinal tract and alleviate the stress and anxiety associated with these issues.

Healing Modalities

Deep relaxation (see page 115)

Visualization (see page 84)

Water (see page 66)

Yoga (see pages 58–59)

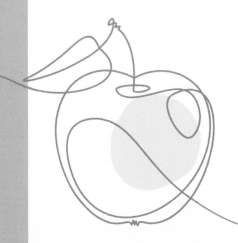

Physiological Genetic Disorders

Muscular Dystrophy (MD), Amyotrophic Lateral Sclerosis (ALS)

Muscular dystrophy encompasses a variety of genetically inherited diseases that over time cause varying degrees of skeletal- and muscle-tissue breakdown. This results in a progressive weakening of the muscles and can lead to an impairment of the use of the arms and legs. ALS has a similar effect, but is mainly neurological in nature and may progress to full immobilization and an inability to speak.

Developing a daily meditation practice can greatly enhance the quality of life for those affected by these degenerative and incurable diseases. Visualization and mindfulness meditation can reduce stress and cultivate feelings of wellbeing. Also, breathing techniques can help energize and relax the mind, alleviating depression, anxiety, and feelings of despair. Because the mind, vision, and hearing are usually not affected by either of these diseases, having tools that primarily utilize guided imagery and breathing techniques can be of great benefit.

Healing Modalities

Breathing (see page 64)
Meditation (see pages 82–87)
Visualization (see page 84)

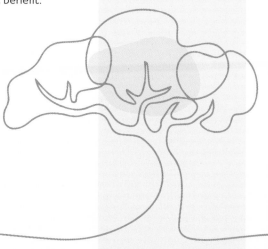

Physiological Neurological Ailments

Multiple Sclerosis (MS), Peripheral Neuropathy

Diseases of the nervous system impede the flow of electrical impulses, resulting in incomplete, disrupted, or blocked communication from one part of the body to another. When the energetic signals are not being transferred effectively, pain, numbness, dysfunction of movement, or the impairment of sensation or cognition may be the result.

Having an awareness of how energy flows through the body allows for conscious intervention with breathing techniques, visualization, and meditation practices that can facilitate an experience of this energy flow.

Healing Modalities

Qigong (see page 49)
Yoga (see pages 58–59)

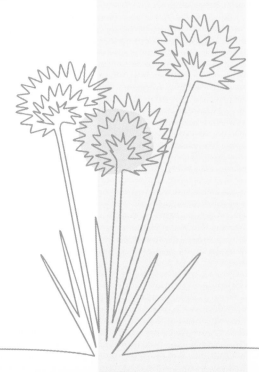

Physiological Blood Disorders

Diabetes—Type 2

The pancreas is an organ that secretes the hormone insulin to metabolize glucose and make energy available to the body's cells and tissues. However, excessive blood sugar levels, caused by obesity or chronic stress, can lead to type-2 diabetes as a result of damage to the pancreas that decreases its ability to produce insulin. This results in chronically high blood sugar levels which can lead to serious issues with the cardiovascular system and the capillaries in the kidneys, eyes, and peripheral nerves.

Conscious eating and stress reduction can help to improve the body's ability to balance blood sugar levels and minimize the effects of type-2 diabetes.

Healing Modalities

Deep relaxation (see page 115)

Meditation (see pages 82–87)

Physiological Sleeping Disorders

Insomnia, Sleep Apnea, Restless Legs Syndrome

Many sleep-related disorders are associated with breathing difficulties caused by underlying stress. Learning how to optimize your breathing can facilitate stimulation of the parasympathetic nervous system or deep relaxation and provide efficient oxygen transfer in the lungs.

Having a practice that includes proper breathing techniques will strengthen the diaphragm and abdominal muscles, so that a level of relaxation can be achieved to provide deep, restful, and healing sleep.

Healing Modalities

Breathing (see page 64)

Deep relaxation (see page 115)

Meditation (see pages 82–87)

Visualization (see page 84)

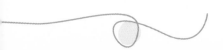

Physiological

Cancer

A variety of cancers cause the uncontrolled and abnormal growth of cells. This can lead to a critical disruption of the body's systems and structures. Meditation and visualization techniques can greatly increase the quality of life for people suffering from cancer, as well as the debilitating side effects of cancer treatments. Also, improving your diet will provide your body with the nutrients it needs to heal itself and diminish the energy needed to balance the effects of an unhealthy diet. Foods to include are unprocessed, organic, fresh meat and vegetables. You should also reduce the consumption of processed foods, especially those that contain salt and refined sugar.

In the face of this extremely challenging illness, having a daily practice that focuses on maintaining a healthy mind and body through conscious eating and energy balancing can facilitate feelings of relief and have a calming effect.

Healing Modalities

Breathing (see page 64)
Meditation (see pages 82–87)
Visualization (see page 84)

Physiological

Osteoporosis

Increased porosity of bone tissue, usually in the elderly, can result in fractures of the hips, legs, pelvis, and vertebrae. Conscious eating and an awareness of proper musculoskeletal alignment can help to ensure that energy and weight transfer occur efficiently and optimally.

Developing a practice that includes load-bearing exercises can help to increase bone density and minimize brittle and weak bones.

Healing Modalities

Qigong (see page 49)
Yoga (see pages 58–59)

Physiological

Chronic Fatigue Syndrome (CFS), Fibromyalgia

Chronic fatigue syndrome and fibromyalgia are difficult to diagnose and treat with Western medicine. The associated anxiety, depression, exhaustion, and insomnia that result from chronic and severe fatigue, along with physical pain, can be debilitating and make it very challenging to live a productive and satisfying life. Energizing the system and reducing stress may help with chronic fatigue. Similarly, focusing our attention toward thoughts of calm and wellbeing may help mitigate the pain.

Following a lifestyle that includes energetic practices which stimulate the sympathetic nervous system will energize the body and help those suffering from chronic fatigue. Similarly, energetic practices that stimulate the parasympathetic nervous system will relax the body and may also diminish the pain of fibromyalgia. These practices can also provide relief from the anxiety and depression caused by both chronic fatigue and fibromyalgia.

Healing Modalities

Breathing (see page 64)
Qigong (see page 49)
The Five Tibetan Rites (see pages 108–113)

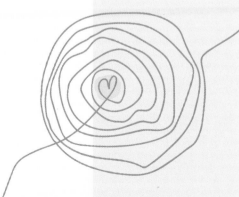

Psychological Ailments

Ailments, disorders, and diseases related to psychological, emotional, or spiritual imbalances can be addressed using a variety of energy movement, release, and processing techniques. EFT (tapping), meditation, and breathing techniques assist in facilitating the flow of energy throughout the body, and can remove blockages as well as provide relief and freedom from past traumas. They can also be useful in processing ongoing trauma and avoiding the reactivation of upsetting issues from the past.

Psychological Behavioral Disorders

Obsessive Compulsive Disorder (OCD) and Attention Deficit Hyperactivity Disorder (ADHD)

OCD and ADHD are similar in that they are both thought to be the result of hormonal imbalances in the secretion of specific neurotransmitters such as serotonin, dopamine, and norepinephrine. These conditions have similar causes and effects. Both OCD and ADHD may involve both behavioral and mental imbalances that present as anxiety around the perception of a lack of control or the avoidance of clutter and disorganization, as well as an inability to focus attention on a task. Making connections with others that have similar life experiences may help to alleviate these types of behavioral imbalances.

Healing Modalities

Breathing (see page 64)

Deep relaxation (see page 115)

Meditation (see pages 82–87)

Visualization (see page 84)

Psychological Eating Disorders

Bulimia and Anorexia Nervosa

Obsessions around food, body weight, and body shape could be influenced by genetic, psychological, or social factors. However, a foundation for healing can be created by cultivating deep emotional connections with people, focusing on similarities rather than differences, and strengthening the belief that nothing is wrong or needs to be fixed.

With this foundation and support from a mental health professional, a regular practice of healthy self-awareness and self-perception can be developed. This can be of great benefit for treating eating disorders and can reinforce a goal of a healthy body, rather than a body that matches some ideal promoted by society.

Healing Modalities

Meditation (see pages 82–87)

Qigong (see page 49)

Yoga (see pages 58–59)

Psychological Mental Illness Disorders

Bipolar Disease (manic-depressive disorder), Borderline Personality Disorder (BPD), Post Traumatic Stress Disorder (PTSD), Body Dysmorphic Disorder (BDD)

Minimizing stress using energy-balancing exercises can be beneficial in mitigating the challenges presented by serious mental illness. In addition to balancing energy, decreasing stress using parasympathetic stimulating exercises may also be helpful if these are included as part of a regular mental health program.

Healing Modalities

Breathing (see page 64)

Deep relaxation (see page 115)

Meditation (see pages 82–87)

Visualization (see page 84)

Psychological Mood Disorders

Anxiety/Depression

Persistent and excessive anxiety and depression are often related to chronic stress and to feelings of uncertainty and a lack of control. They may also be related to past or current trauma or persistent situational events. Having tools that activate the energetic body to balance blockages or imbalances can be beneficial in mitigating the emotional ups and downs of anxiety and depression.

Healing Modalities

Breathing (see page 64)
Deep relaxation (see page 115)
Qigong (see page 49)
Tai chi (see page 50)
Yoga (see pages 58–59)

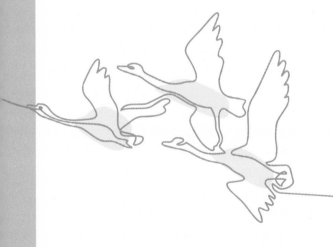

Psychological Social Energy Fields

Parties, Family Gatherings, Teaching, Leading Meetings

Having an awareness of the energy in a social environment greatly enhances the quality of your communication and connection to those who are listening. Cultivating a variety of relationships with others can help you adapt to certain situations, and offers a specific way to communicate within each type of relationship. Both the way you listen and the way you speak can be influenced by the quality of the energy in your communication.

Heart-centered awareness that includes gratitude, empathy, and compassion for others will provide the healing energy needed for deep connection and authenticity. Having a daily practice of energy exercises that keeps you present and connected will provide you with the balance and power needed for optimal communication and increase the likelihood that what you are offering will be effectively received.

Healing Modalities

Breathing (see page 64)
Meditation (see pages 82–87)

Visualization (see page 84)

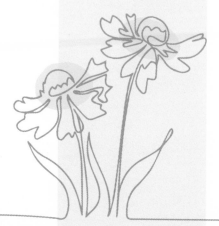

Mechanical Ailments

Mechanical imbalances often involve a misalignment of the skeletal system or imbalances in the skeletal muscles. Strain and injuries can result in inflammation of the soft and connective tissue in and around joints, tendons, and ligaments which allow for the smooth and balanced mechanical movement of the body. Having an awareness of how energy fields affect inflammation and alignment can help to mitigate the inflammation that leads to these mechanical issues.

Mechanical Connective Tissue

Plantar Fasciitis, Arthritis, Carpal Tunnel Syndrome (CTS)

Persistent, repetitive motion of any of the joints can lead to irritation, and eventually inflammation, of connective tissue. Plantar fasciitis is caused by the inflammation of the connective tissue on the sole of the foot, which results in pain in the heel and below the arch of the foot. Carpal tunnel syndrome is caused by a repetitive motion of the fingers which can lead to inflammation of the tendons in the wrist.

Finger qigong, toe qigong, and hand *mudras* can help to facilitate the flow of energy through the hands and feet, and also maintain the range of motion in the joints of the hands, wrists, feet, and ankles.

Healing Modalities

Meditation (see pages 82–87)

Qigong (see page 49)

Yoga (see pages 58–59)

Mechanical Skeletal Alignment Disorders

Neck, Shoulders, Elbows, Wrists, Fingers, Upper Back, Lower Back, Sacroiliac Joints, Hips, Knees, Ankles, Toes

All the joints of the body involve an interface of some type of connective tissue and supporting ligaments and tendons. When the body is properly aligned and balanced, it is able to distribute the forces of gravity and any loads imposed upon it. Proper balance keeps the muscles and joints working in concert to provide mobility and efficiently move us through the world. When there is chronic strain, torque, extreme loads, or physical blunt-force trauma, the musculoskeletal system can be thrown out of balance and, over the long term, this can cause problems that compromise our ability to remain ambulatory and function in the physical world. Understanding how bodily energies and forces work can help raise awareness of how to use our bodies in an optimal way.

Having an understanding of the natural flow of energy that occurs when we sit, stand, walk, run, lift, or jump helps when practicing exercises that promote aligned and balanced musculoskeletal movement.

Healing Modalities

Qigong (see page 49)
Tai chi (see page 50)
Yoga (see pages 58–59)

CHAPTER 3
THE ENERGY HEALING ARTS

In this chapter, you will find an overview of many different energy healing modalities, with wide-ranging benefits. Each modality includes an at-a-glance information list so you can find the method most suited to address your concern.

MOVEMENT THERAPIES
Martial Arts, Massage, Yoga, & Dance

Movement therapies include any of the martial arts, massage techniques, and most forms of yoga and dance. In each of these modalities the movement of energy through the body is experienced as a flow or wave of changing color, light, temperature, texture, or feeling. Key to understanding the energetic aspects of each therapy is visualizing the toric field of your body and even the toric field of the practitioner. When the body is in healthy flow, physically and energetically, the body's electromagnetic field follows the dynamic flow in the vibrant field of the torus.

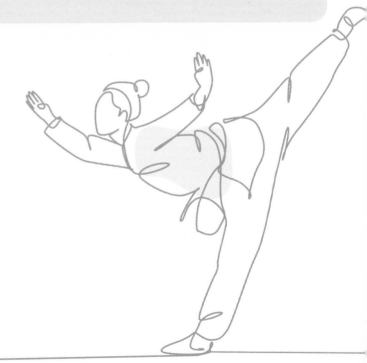

Having an awareness of the direction and flow of chi moving through the body will help guide the movements of qigong.

Martial Arts

Many of the martial arts have traditionally provided a way to cultivate and direct chi, to facilitate the optimum flow of energy through the body's toric field. Using conscious awareness of the body and mind, the martial artist is not only able to control and direct his own energetic flow, but also to influence the energetic flow of others. Whether it is tai chi, qigong, aikido, jujitsu, or kung fu, the common denominator in these martial arts is a conscious awareness of the body's position in space and time (proprioception) and the presence of a flow of energy through, away from, and toward the body.

Qigong

Proficiency Level: ●
(Beginners start here)
Practitioner Support:
Independent/Instructor
Benefits:
Relaxing, Energizing, Focusing, Balancing, Awareness
Equipment Required:
None

The ancient practice of qigong (*chee gung* or *ki gung*) literally means life energy (*chi*) cultivation (*gung*). It has been practiced in China since 300BCE to encourage the movement of chi via the meridian channels (which are also used in acupuncture). Like many wellness modalities, qigong helps to reduce stress and promote relaxation, to facilitate the body's innate ability to heal itself.

Using gentle, flowing movements, qigong practice seeks to awaken and cultivate chi to balance and harmonize the life energy force in and around the body. With practice, it is possible to perceive small shifts of energy which helps to focus the effort to release blocked energy and facilitate the flow of chi.

Tai Chi

Proficiency Level: ● ●
Practitioner Support:
Independent/Instructor
Benefits:
Strengthening, Awareness,
Connecting, Flexibility
Equipment Required:
None

Tai chi (*taiji*) is most closely translated as "supreme ultimate" and originated as a form of martial art. Note that the chi portion of the name should not be confused with the chi defined as "life energy." The term "tai chi" conceptualizes the flux or energetic flow between yin and yang, and may be considered to be a more complex form of qigong.

Tai chi uses coordinated focus on the body, the breath, and the mind to balance the yin and yang energies through an extensive series of movements to achieve connection to the "supreme ultimate." Because of the difficulty of learning the long sequences of the original form, short forms have been developed to make the practice more accessible to beginners.

Throughout tai chi sequences, energy flow is felt or seen moving through and around the body. The movements follow the flow of the energetic toric field to balance, enhance, or strengthen the field in order to bring vitality and flexibility to both body and mind.

Although tai chi is slow and gentle and doesn't leave you breathless, it can build strength and flexibility in both body and mind.

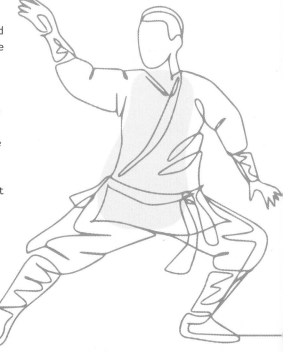

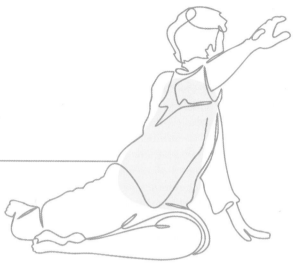

By understanding the biomechanics of body movement we can re-educate the body so that it can flow through space and time smoothly and in harmony with itself and its environment.

Feldenkrais

Proficiency Level: ● ● ●
Practitioner Support:
Independent/Instructor
Benefits:
Harmony, Awareness, Aligning,
Posture, Flexibility
Equipment Required:
None

The Feldenkrais Method was developed by Moshe Feldenkrais as a way of promoting a conscious awareness of how our bodies move. Working with and against the force of gravity, and with the natural push and pull of the tissues of the body, it is possible to bend, extend, flex, and rotate the joints and limbs with conscious awareness.

The proper carriage of the head on the shoulders and the torso on the pelvis enables the development of an intentional, non-habitual way of moving. When we consciously transfer the load from one part of the body to another, our thoughts and sensations are in harmony with our movement.

When we successfully integrate our body movements, we can optimize the efficiency and economy of energy utilization and move with a poised sense of our own royal presence. In this space, we create a dynamic sense of confidence as we move through the world.

Pilates

Proficiency Level: ● ● ●
Practitioner Support:
Independent/Instructor
Benefits:
Flexibility, Balancing,
Strengthening, Aligning
Equipment Required:
None

Pilates is a form of gentle movement exercise developed by Joseph Pilates in the early 1900s. It is performed on a mat or on a specific piece of equipment designed for a Pilates workout. The main distinction between a gym workout and a Pilates workout is that Pilates generally focuses on balanced movements to develop core strength and flexibility.

The basic principles include centering attention on the core of the body between the diaphragm and the pubic bone, focusing the awareness on each movement, controlling the actions being taken with each movement, and performing each movement with precision, fluidity, and conscious breath.

The movements include a holistic approach to biodynamic action, using tension and compression of the muscles, tendons, and bones to move the head, shoulders, arms, spine, hips, and legs in a concerted way, thus providing balanced support and structure to the body (tensegrity).

This physiological, interdependent motion is extended beyond the body energetically and strengthens the electromagnetic field around the body, helping to release blockages and improve the sensitivity of your awareness of your body in the world (proprioception).

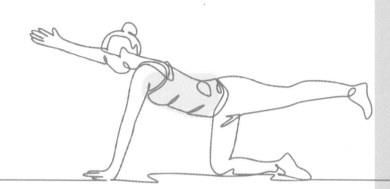

While Pilates training focuses on core strength, it trains the body as an integrated whole.

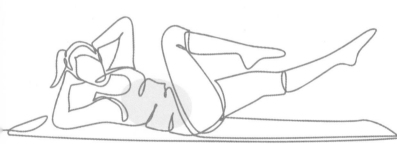

With thousands of possible exercises and modifications, Pilates workouts can be tailored to individual needs and desires.

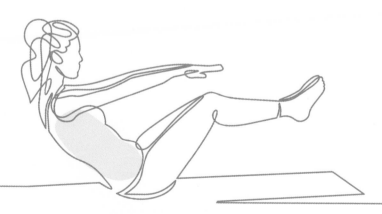

When our core is strong, the frame of the body is supported, leading to improved alignment.

Massage

The direct person-to-person contact of massage therapy greatly facilitates the movement of energy in the client by the therapist. The flow of energy is actually enhanced because of the exchange of energy between the therapist and the client, and often provides immediate relief from pain and discomfort. Because the effects of this therapy are felt so quickly, it is easy to finish the therapy too soon and end up treating the symptoms and skipping the underlying issues that may be causing the pain or discomfort. Therefore, it is beneficial to use massage therapy on a regular basis to stay well after any injury or until an issue has been alleviated.

As an energetic healing modality, massage falls into one of the most mechanical categories of movement medicine. It is well known to many people and there is variety of methods to choose from. There is an abundance of licensed massage therapists to choose from in cities and towns, large and small.

Swedish

Proficiency Level: ● ● ●
Practitioner Support:
Practitioner required
Benefits:
Relaxing, Soothing, Flowing, Opening
Equipment Required:
None

Swedish and deep tissue massages are probably the most well-known types of massage. They definitely have many differences, but one similarity is the goal of facilitating the flow of physical systems as well as the energetic fields of the body.

Swedish massage can release tension, reduce anxiety, and provide deep relaxation to create an overall feeling of wellbeing. By using long, smooth strokes, the therapist encourages the circulation of the blood and the flow of lymph drainage. The circular, kneading strokes can facilitate the softening of muscular tension and an opening up of the joints. Energetically, the movement encouraged by the therapist will provide a sense of flow and expansion.

Deep Tissue

Proficiency Level: ● ● ●
Practitioner Support:
Practitioner required
Benefits:
Healing, Flexibility, Freeing, Releasing
Equipment Required:
None

Deep tissue massage uses strokes and techniques similar to Swedish massage, but it is done using more pressure in order to go deeper into the tissues of the muscles, tendons, and joints. It is primarily geared toward speeding up the healing time for injuries, as well as for the relief of neck, shoulder, back, and joint pain. Overall, deep tissue massage will increase blood flow to areas of concern which, in turn, will reduce inflammation in the affected area.

Energetically, the healing of injuries helps to release energetic blockages so that our electromagnetic fields can flow with freedom and vibrancy.

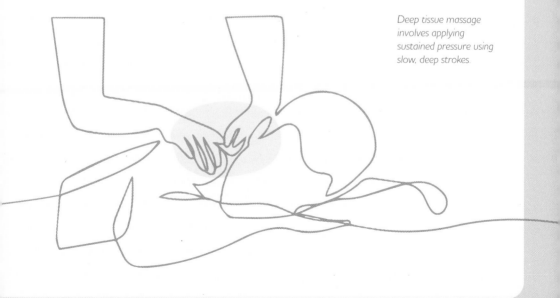

Deep tissue massage involves applying sustained pressure using slow, deep strokes.

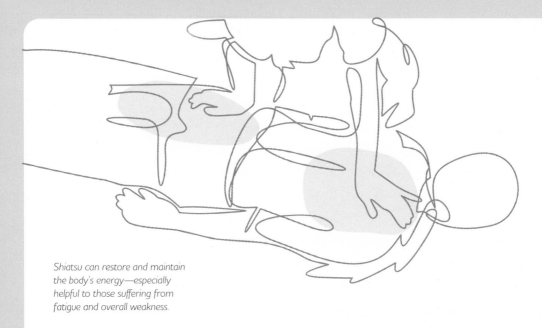

Shiatsu can restore and maintain the body's energy—especially helpful to those suffering from fatigue and overall weakness.

Shiatsu

Proficiency Level: ● ● ●
Practitioner Support:
Practitioner required
Benefits:
Flowing, Opening, Relaxing
Equipment Required:
None

Shiatsu massage was developed from a type of traditional Japanese bodywork called *anma* which translates as "finger pressure." Through a combination of massage techniques that include acupressure and trigger-point release, a shiatsu therapist uses their fingers, knuckles, elbows, knees, and the soles of the feet and palms of the hands to apply rhythmic pressure to precise points and to stretch tissues to facilitate the flow of blood, lymph, and nerve impulses, and also the energetic life force through the body.

The therapist may also place the client in specific positions and use their own body weight to lean into the client to open tight/constricted joints and improve the flow of all body systems.

Thai Yoga

Proficiency Level: ● ● ●
Practitioner Support:
Practitioner required
Benefits:
Mobilizing, Loosening, Opening, Flowing
Equipment Required:
None

Thai yoga massage is a technique that uses assisted yoga postures to pull, stretch, rotate, or apply tension to the limbs, spine, and neck, and, as in shiatsu, the therapist uses parts of their own body as tools for passive joint mobilization.

A Thai yoga therapist tunes into the state of the client and uses gentle rocking motions, various types of stretching movements, and deep breathing to open and release blockages and to facilitate flow through the main energy meridians (also known as sen). The therapist will sense and evaluate the range of movement, determine if any restrictions or tightness exist, and gently push to increase the range of motion and so gently open and release the muscles, tendons, and fascia.

Thai yoga massage improves circulation and lymphatic flow, boosting energy levels and reducing stress.

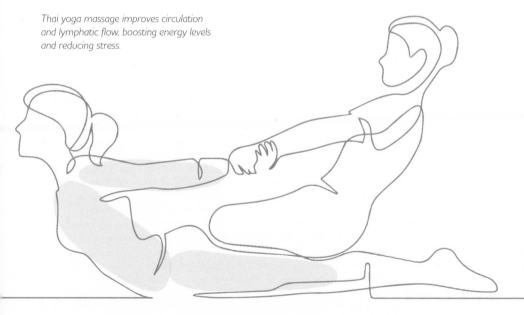

Yoga and Dance

Many types of yoga and dance utilize the body's ability to move dynamically in a variety of positions and in doing so produce an astonishing expression of art through the body. Whether it is kundalini, vinyasa, or Ashtanga yoga, or Sufi, ballet, or ballroom dancing, yoga and dance can provide an effective system of coordinated movement sequences that increases flexibility and releases both physical and energetic blockages. Any physical movements performed with intention and awareness will affect the field of energy that surrounds the body.

Kundalini

Proficiency Level: ● ●
Practitioner Support:
Independent/Instructor
Benefits:
Centering, Grounding, Connecting, Balancing, Flowing, Clearing
Equipment Required:
Yoga mat

Kundalini yoga is a modality that vitalizes and balances the nervous system through coordinated breath and movement. The kundalini sequences (*kriyas*) are performed with specific meditation chanting (*mantras*) and hand/finger poses (*mudras*), which all contribute to the strengthening of the autonomic, central, and peripheral nervous systems. Breathing techniques (*pranayama*) oxygenate and purify the blood and improve circulation which, in turn, helps to reduce inflammation and decrease pain.

Energetically, kundalini yoga extends and strengthens the electromagnetic field of the body and "pushes out" dense energy frequencies or blockages that can impede flow within the toric field. The awareness of kundalini energy moving up and down the spine around the spinal cord is improved with consistent practice. The kriyas are often specific to the seven physical chakras and their corresponding endocrine glands. The regulation of the endocrine system ensures that a proper balance of hormones is achieved and available in any situation, and that the body's systems, organs, and tissues will respond accordingly.

The breathwork within the kriyas is so powerful that it starts to facilitate a release of energetic and physical blockages, leading to a greater sense of self.

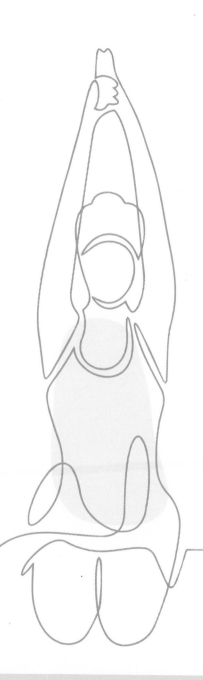

Sufi Spinning Meditation

Proficiency Level: ● ● ●
Practitioner Support:
Independent/Instructor
Benefits:
Awareness, Balancing,
Connecting, Meditative
Equipment Required:
None

The whirling dervishes of the Sufi tradition are an excellent example of how patterns of energetic motion, which are produced by this spinning meditation, can be physically seen. The head, arms, and feet, along with the robe and hat that are worn for this meditation, trace lines while spinning to reveal a beautiful expression of the field of energy around the dancer.

The spinning is done in such a way that the dancer does not get dizzy or lose their balance. Their regular and precise foot placements allow them to slip into a meditative state and disappear into a whirl of energy. The results for the dancer include an expansion of their energetic bodies as well a calm, relaxed sense of self with a deep connection to the universe.

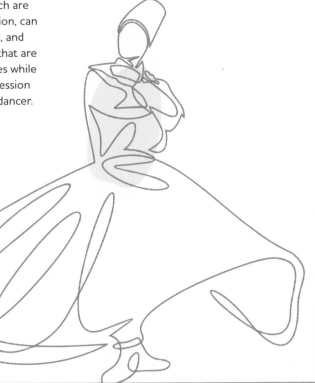

Whether viewed from above or from the side, the shapes produced by the dance are exquisite.

Dance

Proficiency Level: ●
(Beginners start here)
Practitioner Support:
Independent/Instructor/Practitioner
Benefits:
Joyful, Balancing, Coordination,
Precision, Expressive
Equipment Required:
None

Whether it is through partnered dance
or individual dance, the flow of energy
through dance movement produces an
exquisite and dynamic flow that allows
for an expansion of flexibility, extension,
and movement.

The individual dancer can move freely and
spontaneously to music and improvise
the choreography by following the
energetic flow that is being experienced
while listening to music. The ability to
sense whether the sound is expanding
or contracting will naturally lead to a
corresponding pulse of energy which is
often seen in modern dance.

All partner dancing, although often
structured and precise, requires a keen
sense of proprioception of each dancer
as an individual as well as combined,
focused, coordinated movements,
including spinning, pivoting, lifting, and
holding. The dance movements are
performed in synchrony with millisecond
timing and precision, thus producing a
physical expression of the music and an
overlapping of two individual toric fields
into a larger and more powerful torus.

*The intellectual disciplines of learning a
dance and training the body to move
as the mind dictates induces discipline
in all one does.*

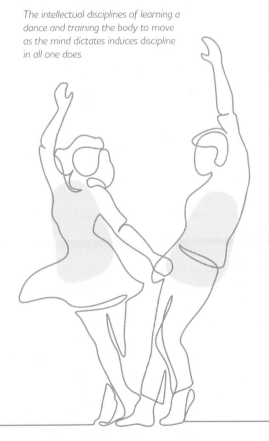

ENERGY FLOW THERAPIES
Earth, Air, Water

The human body exists in an electrical field of positive and negative charges which create potential for energy flow across various boundaries. Everything from cell membranes, tissue bundles, and the organs themselves is affected by these gradients of potential energy. Whether the gradients exist through air (such as lightning discharges), earth (ionic potential gradients through the feet/hands), or water (electrolyte absorption), or through the skin (Epsom salt baths, ocean water), the natural homeostatic process will balance the charges in the body to optimize health.

Nerve impulses are initiated by action potentials across cell membranes and cause depolarization to allow a signal to travel in a specific direction from neuron to neuron. Ions of $Ca+$, $K+$, $Na+$, and $Mg+$ all play an important role in regulating the electrical balance of energy throughout the body.

Earth

Grounding

Proficiency Level: ●
(*Beginners start here*)
Practitioner Support:
Independent
Benefits:
Grounding, Balancing, Flowing, Relaxing
Equipment Required:
None

The polarity of positive and negative charges can be affected by grounding yourself energetically to the Earth's naturally occurring ionic potential gradients. Walking barefoot on the grass or directly on the earth can affect the balance of your energetic body, which in turn helps to systemically reduce inflammation, thus facilitating the body's innate healing ability.

This balancing or grounding can help to create a balanced electrical field which may facilitate healing and lead to an overall sense of wellbeing. The

balancing of electrolytes throughout the body provides the electrical gradients needed for energetic flow within cellular organelles, flow across membranes, between cells and tissues, and throughout the nervous system. Incorporating grounding as part of a daily practice can contribute to a healthy lifestyle.

In addition to outdoor barefoot grounding, an indoor grounding mat placed on the floor, with bare feet resting on the mat, can also be used. You can also use a larger grounding mat which is placed on a bed for sleeping on. These methods actually connect you to the electric field of the Earth through a physical grounding wire.

When skin comes into contact with the ground, the human body soaks up negatively-charged electrons from the earth.

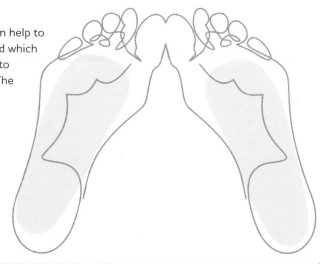

Air

Breathing Techniques

Proficiency Level: ● ●
Practitioner Support:
Independent/Instructor
Benefits:
Energizing, Calming, Healing, Flowing
Equipment Required:
None

Breathing is one of the most unconscious actions performed by humans. We can sleep, work, and play without giving much thought to our breath. Ironically, it is the one process that we cannot do without for more than a few seconds, or perhaps a few minutes after some practice. We can go weeks with little or no food, days with little or no water, but air is essential to life.

Some types of yoga utilize specific breathing techniques (*pranayama*) to affect the yogic practice. The techniques utilize a preset pattern (such as inhale, inhale, inhale, exhale) to count the number of in- and out-breaths in order to produce different energetic results.

For slow, deep breathing, air is drawn in through the nose as the belly is softened and allowed to be pushed out by the diaphragm; then, on the exhale, the navel is pulled back toward the spine by the abdominal muscles as air is slowly released through the mouth. Other patterns include a smooth inhale through the nose over a specified count and pausing the breath for a specified count, which is then followed by a smooth exhale through the mouth for a specified count. These breathing techniques can induce parasympathetic responses that lower the respiration rate, heart rate, and blood pressure, resulting in decreased stress and a feeling of deep relaxation.

Some of the flow or vinyasa yogic practices utilize ujjayi breathing, which slows the rate of respiration and facilitates deep relaxation. Ujjayi breath involves slow, deep breathing, inhaling and exhaling through the nose. The throat is somewhat constricted, which produces a rasping sound as air passes over the glottis at the top of the bronchial tube. To practice ujjayi breathing, focus on allowing your ribs to expand laterally on the inhale, rather than allowing the diaphragm to push the belly out. This has a calming effect, and increases the oxygenation of the blood and the internal body temperature. The practice is used to cultivate pranic energy and increase overall stamina.

"Breath of Fire" is done in some yogic practices (for example, kundalini yoga) to energize and stimulate the nervous system. This technique uses a series of

short in- and out-breaths, taken very
quickly through the nose, to oxygenate
the blood, increase circulation, and
expand the energetic field of the body.
The technique is usually practiced
while holding a specific yoga pose for
a short duration.

*Breathing consciously
can produce
extraordinary changes
in the body's systems,
which can be both
stimulating and relaxing.*

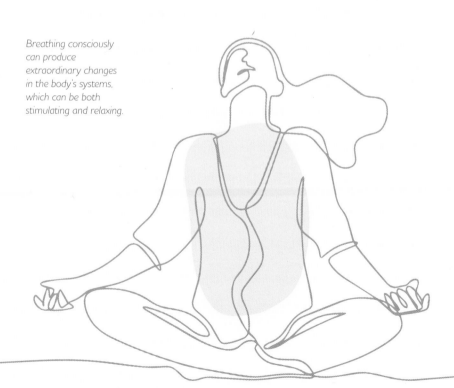

Water

Absorption

Proficiency Level: ●
(Beginners start here)
Practitioner Support:
Independent
Benefits:
Nurturing, Connecting, Healing,
Balancing, Flowing
Equipment Required:
None

People around the world use the waters
of the oceans and seas, natural mineral
hot springs, and sacred rivers such as the
Ganges to help heal sickness or injury
and maintain health. Ocean water is
beneficial because it has a very similar
chemical composition to the plasma of
human blood. Sacred rivers encompass the
pranic energy of the river itself along with
the field of energy created by the people
who visit the site.

Chemically, the molecular structure of
water is such that it can provide the
basis for organic chemical reactions and
electrical currents, enabling the body to
function properly. Complex organic life,
as we know it, cannot exist without water.

Because of the amazing porosity of the
skin, water and its constituents are readily
absorbed and are made available to the
body. Whether water is drunk or absorbed
through the skin, it can facilitate ionic
electrolyte balance, nutrient absorption in
the intestines, and general hydration for
the proper metabolism of cells, tissues,
organs, and the interstitial spaces of
connective tissue.

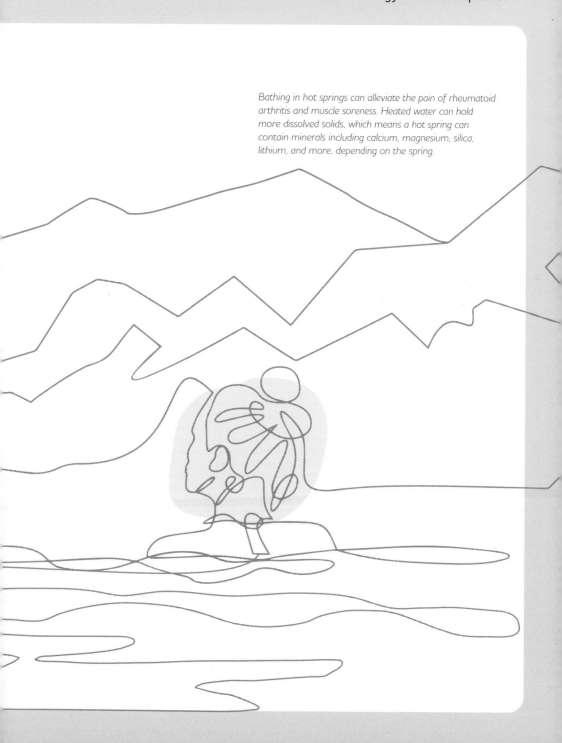

Bathing in hot springs can alleviate the pain of rheumatoid arthritis and muscle soreness. Heated water can hold more dissolved solids, which means a hot spring can contain minerals including calcium, magnesium, silica, lithium, and more, depending on the spring.

BIOENERGETIC THERAPIES
Hands-off, Hands-on

A number of therapies can be used to directly affect the bioenergetic fields of the body. Some therapies, such as crystal healing and Biofield Tuning, are performed without physical touch; others such as reflexology or acupressure affect the energy fields by gentle touching of parts of the body. For some of these types of therapies, a trained/certified practitioner is needed to affect the energy field.

Energy manipulation therapies depend on a focused intention combined with a sensitivity of perception to detect types of energy and changes in energy as the therapy is being practiced. For these types of therapies, there is a sense of quieting the mind and the body, and "stepping aside" to allow perception of a field of energy. It is often helpful to practice some of the hands-off therapies first in order to inform the type of hands-on therapy to use to affect the bioenergetic field.

Hands-off

Crystal Medicine

Proficiency Level: ●
(Beginners start here)
Practitioner Support:
Independent/Practitioner
Benefits:
Balancing, Healing, Releasing, Freeing
Equipment Required:
Relevant crystals/gems

Crystals can be placed on the body, worn as jewelry, or carried in pouches so that you can receive the benefits of their specific energetic frequencies. They can be used to clear dense energy and absorb negative energy in a particular space, balance chakras, and balance and remove energetic blockages in the physical body as well as the emotional body. The subtle energy generated by crystals often has specific frequencies of color, light, and sound that correspond to the particular types of crystals. Their effectiveness is greatly influenced by your intention and knowledge of their power.

The chakras are energetic vortexes that correspond to neural plexuses located in different parts of the body along the spine and in the skull. Balanced chakras have a significant influence on the endocrine glands which regulate the release of hormones. These affect many aspects of the body's ability to maintain health through metabolic processes and results in a feeling of overall wellbeing.

A crystal therapist will place healing crystals on or around a client to help unblock, focus, and direct energy.

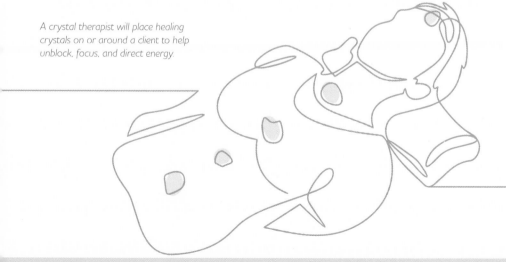

Aromatherapy

Proficiency Level: ●
(*Beginners start here*)
Practitioner Support:
Independent/Practitioner
Benefits:
Calming, Blissful, Healing,
Balancing, Energizing
Equipment Required:
Therapeutic-grade essential oils

Aromatic oils were used medicinally thousands of years ago in Egypt, China, India, Greece, Rome, and Persia, and are more recently being widely used in the West for aromatherapy. These highly concentrated oils are extracted using various methods from different parts of medicinal plants and from their resins.

Specific essential oils can be used in combination with energy therapies such as crystal energy healing and Reiki subtle energy therapy to enhance their therapeutic effects. The highly volatile oils can be used for chakra balancing and to stimulate both sympathetic and parasympathetic responses. Topically

applying oils at points on the body that correspond to a particular chakra, or inhaling the volatile vapors of diffused oils, can produce remarkable energetic and healing effects.

Some of the most powerful essential oils in common use include lavender, peppermint, ginger, clove, cinnamon, frankincense, rosemary, eucalyptus, and melaleuca (tea tree) oil. Peppermint, tea tree, and eucalyptus oils can cool the body and stimulate a sympathetic energetic response almost immediately, promoting a feeling of alertness and clarity. Using frankincense, clove, and ginger oils can warm the body and quickly stimulate a parasympathetic energetic response, promoting a feeling of soothing calmness and relaxation.

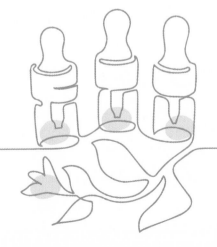

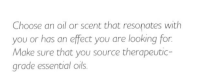
Choose an oil or scent that resonates with you or has an effect you are looking for. Make sure that you source therapeutic-grade essential oils.

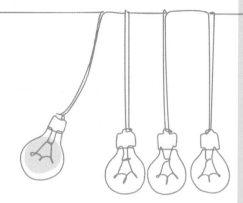

Pendulums help in promoting spiritual and physical healing by locating energetic blocks. They are tools that help in balancing, healing, and clearing both mind and body.

Energy Meters

Proficiency Level: ● ●
Practitioner Support:
Independent/Instructor/Practitioner
Benefits:
Awareness, Balancing,
Energizing, Recalibrating
Equipment Required:
Weighted pendulum, tuning
forks, dowsing rods

Tools for divination are used to identify energetic fields, including the chakras of the body. Dowsing rods have been employed for centuries as a tool for divining the location of water, oil, minerals, or tunnels beneath the surface of the Earth. More recently, pendulums are being used in a similar way to divine or detect changes in energetic fields around the body. A pendulum consists of a string or chain with a weighted stone or object hanging from one end. The string is held in one hand and the weighted end is allowed to hang freely above the body.

Pendulums can be used to perform chakra balancing by detecting underactive or overactive chakras and then recalibrating a particular chakra energy vortex to bring it back into balance. An experienced practitioner can use a pendulum to detect or identify energetic blockages at various locations around the body, and may also be able to determine the direction of energetic flow. This information is helpful and means that the practitioner can then attempt to release, adjust, or balance any chakras or misaligned energetic fields.

Tuning forks are used to detect the boundaries of the body's energetic field and to determine any energetic imbalances in that field. This technique is called Biofield Tuning. The method can be part of a chakra-balancing protocol as well as a method for recalibrating the energetic field.

Hands-on

Reflexology

Proficiency Level: ● ●
Practitioner Support:
Independent/Practitioner
Benefits:
Healing, Calming, Flowing, Relaxing, Stimulating, Energizing
Equipment Required:
None

Reflexology uses a variety of reflex techniques on "body maps" on the soles of the feet, the palms of the hands, and the outer ears to stimulate nerve endings that correspond to different parts of the body. Energetically, reflexology uses the nervous system to increase circulation at specific locations throughout the body which, in turn, facilitates flow in the circulatory, lymph, and nervous systems as well as in the gastrointestinal system.

Energetic blockages, as well as physical blockages, occur when the normal flow of systems is reduced, resulting in a diminished delivery of nutrients and the reduced elimination of waste and the by-products of metabolism from cells and tissues. Increasing circulation to organs and tissues helps to facilitate the body's ability to provide more nutrients for the proper functioning of various systems and to remove toxins, thus preventing disease, inflammation, or infection.

Specific reflex points are used either to energize the body or to relax and calm it. By focusing on specific organs/glands, reflexology can stimulate the production of hormones and elicit a sympathetic or parasympathetic response to improve the availability of energy or to reduce anxiety to slow and balance frenetic energy, respectively.

With repeated pressure and manipulation of nerve endings, reflexology can help to clear any channels of blocked energy.

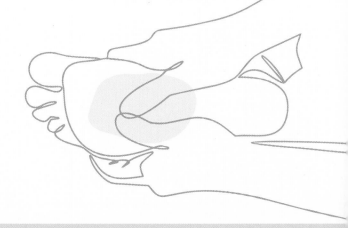

Jin Shin Jyutsu

Proficiency Level: ● ●
Practitioner Support:
Independent/Practitioner
Benefits:
Calming, Healing, Stillness, Flow, Releasing
Equipment Required:
None

Jin Shin Jyutsu is a form of light touch therapy, similar to acupressure, which uses gentle finger pressure on specific points of the body to facilitate the flow of physical and energetic systems. Literally translated as "The Art of the Creator Through the Person of Knowing Compassion," Jin Shin Jyutsu seeks to harmonize and restore balance to the energy or chi of the body.

By squeezing the fingers of each hand, each of which corresponds to the emotions of worry, fear, anger, grief, and pretense, or by applying pressure to a specific series of energy lock points,

known as the 26 "Safety Energy Locks," Jin Shin Jyutsu therapy can facilitate the release of physical or energetic blocks or stagnation and open up pathways for the overall wellbeing of the body.

The process of moving energy in the body may help to reduce stress and enhance feelings of deep relaxation and calm stillness. It may also result in the reduction of physical or emotional pain or discomfort, facilitate the proper nourishment of the cells, tissues, and organs, and help balance overall energetic flow throughout the body.

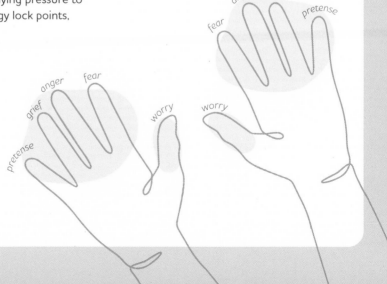

Polarity Therapy

Proficiency Level: ● ● ●
Practitioner Support:
Practitioner required
Benefits:
Balancing, Stillness, Flowing,
Healing, Nourishing, Nurturing
Equipment Required:
None

Polarity therapy is an energy medicine that provides a holistic approach to balancing the physical, mental, emotional, and spiritual aspects of living. Energy is the basis of all of these aspects. It incorporates diet and nutrition, physical exercise and bodywork, and meditation and prayer. Unlike Reiki, which draws energy from external sources, polarity therapy works with the energy currents within the body.

This subtle energy practice balances the positive and negative poles of the electromagnetic field of the body. The electromagnetic currents of energy flow back and forth from the head to the toes, left side to right side, and front to back through the body. These currents can be impeded or resisted by physiological or energetic disharmony caused by stress, unhealthy lifestyles, or injury. The blocked or weakened flow of energy diminishes the optimum function of cells, tissues, organs, and systems, and may lead to various issues or diseases.

The polarity therapist's goal is to rebalance the flow by opening the energy blocks to release the stagnant energy and thus restore the electrical balance to the energy fields and currents of the body. By placing the hands on a particular location along the chakras and meridians of the body, polarity therapy practitioners can feel or "see" where the energy flow is blocked and assist in releasing or removing the block and restoring energetic flow to the area being worked on. Once the electrical system has been balanced, the energetic flow can then, in turn, facilitate the circulation of the blood as well as lymphatic and neurologic flow, and so greatly assist the body's innate ability to heal itself.

Polarity therapy is focused on reestablishing the balance of the body's natural energy flow, which in turn allows healing to take place.

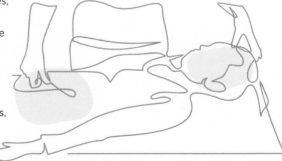

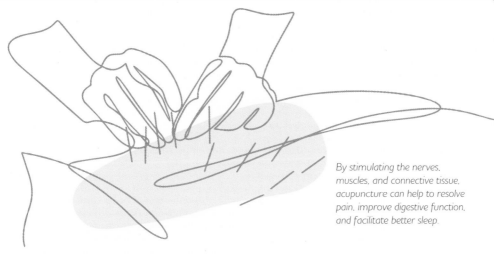

By stimulating the nerves, muscles, and connective tissue, acupuncture can help to resolve pain, improve digestive function, and facilitate better sleep.

Acupuncture

Proficiency Level: ● ● ●
Practitioner Support:
Practitioner required
Benefits:
Healing, Relieving, Flowing, Clearing, Stimulating
Equipment Required:
None

Acupuncture originated 3,000 years ago as part of Traditional Chinese Medicine (TCM) to treat a number of issues and diseases. Very thin needles are used to stimulate points along the energy pathways (known as meridians) of the body. The general aim of acupuncture is to remove energetic blockages along the meridians to encourage the flow of chi or life energy within the body. This modality differs from many of the other energy medicine techniques in that it requires state licensure, is invasive, and is often covered by insurance.

The acupuncturist uses a number of needles to pierce the skin and stimulate nerves just below the surface. The needles are precisely inserted at meridian points which are selected by the acupuncturist for the specific issue being addressed. The needles remain inserted for anywhere from 15 minutes to an hour, and are carefully removed at the conclusion of the acupuncture session. Acupuncture is known to stimulate the immune system, as well as the gastrointestinal, nervous, endocrine, and cardiovascular systems, and has few known side effects. It can alleviate pain from injury, disease, or stress, and the release of energetic stagnation can lead to feelings of deep relaxation, improved sleep, and a sense of overall wellbeing.

Craniosacral Therapy

Proficiency Level: ● ● ●
Practitioner Support:
Practitioner required
Benefits:
Stillness, Relaxing, Healing, Aligning, Calming, Nurturing, Releasing
Equipment Required:
None

An osteopathic physician named John Upledger pioneered and developed craniosacral therapy in the 1970s. Through his practice of osteopathy, he noticed that the system which maintains the central nervous system (CNS) is well organized and can be influenced by subtle pressure applied by the fingertips and the hands of a practitioner.

The cerebrospinal fluid that surrounds the brain and the spinal cord is encased in a dural membrane that separates the CNS from the circulatory system of the blood and is surrounded by the bones of the skull and the spinal column all the way down to the coccyx. The dural membrane also allows nerves to exit the CNS at points along each of the vertebrae of the spine to innervate the rest of the body.

Because the craniosacral system does not form a circular circuit, it depends on a cranial rhythm to move the cerebrospinal fluid up and down the spine. The subtle flexing of the spine and the small, but perceptible motion of the plates of the cranium create this energetic cranial rhythm.

The so-called "fixed joints" of the sutures in the skull are actually composed of connective tissue that locks the plates together and creates a protective helmet when sudden pressure occurs from a blow to the head. However, when subtle pressure is applied, the sutures are more fluid and allow the plates and bones of the skull to extend and flex, creating a small difference in pressure. This small pressure change helps to move the cerebrospinal fluid, generated in the central ventricles of the brain, down the dural tube in a spiral motion toward the sacrum. At the bottom of the dural tube, surrounded by the sacrum, the fluid changes direction and spirals back up around the spinal cord and to the brain where it is reabsorbed back into the blood's circulatory system.

Craniosacral therapy uses subtle touch techniques to perceive small movements of the dural tube, skull, and spine, and gentle pressure is then applied to various points to help move the cerebrospinal fluid up and down the spine. While deeply connected to the client, the practitioner will attempt to unwind any portions of the dural tube along the spine that appear to be stuck or twisted. Unwinding the craniosacral system will help restore an unimpeded flow of cerebrospinal fluid and alleviate any pressure on nerves that leave the CNS at each vertebra to create an optimal environment for a healthy CNS.

During the session the craniosacral therapist will also attempt to produce a state of "still point" which stimulates a parasympathetic response, resulting in deep relaxation. This still-point state greatly influences the overall energetic flow of all of the body's energetic systems to promote deep healing.

Craniosacral therapy is a hands-on technique that uses gentle touch to examine movement of the membranes and fluids in and around the central nervous system to release tension in the body.

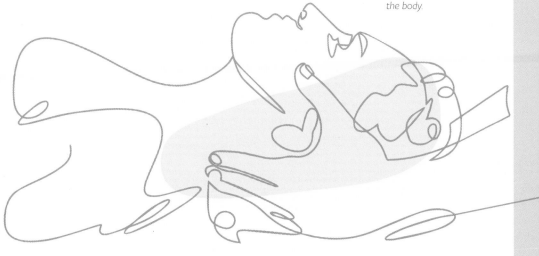

EFT (Emotional Freedom Technique)—Tapping

Proficiency Level: ●
(Beginners start here)
Practitioner Support:
Independent/Instructor
Benefits:
Relieving, Calming, Peaceful,
Freeing, Recalibrating
Equipment Required:
None

The Emotional Freedom Technique (EFT) has been referred to as energy psychology and can be used to create new neural pathways to alleviate both psychological and physical issues. This energy healing modality employs a percussive technique, which involves using the fingertips to tap on the endpoints of the meridians located on the cranial and facial bones of the skull, on and just below the clavicles, and just below the axilla or armpits. The tapping is often accompanied by mantra-like acknowledgments and affirmations of wellness which are associated with an emotion that corresponds to a particular psychological or physical issue.

The process begins with the identification of the issue needing to be addressed. Then, based on the particular issue, an EFT point(s) is chosen for the session. Once the tapping has begun there is a verbal acknowledgment of the emotion being experienced in the present moment because of the issue. This is followed by an affirmation of the imagined feeling or emotion that is desired once the issue has been resolved.

This energy medicine can address feelings of physical pain or emotional distress from psychological issues such as guilt, shame, anger, and resentments from past emotional or physical trauma. The resulting relief from these blockages can facilitate the goal of emotional freedom from suffering.

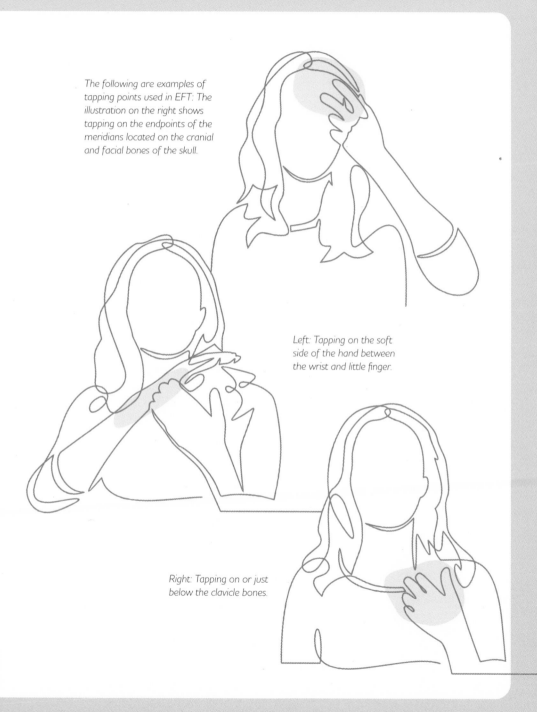

The following are examples of tapping points used in EFT: The illustration on the right shows tapping on the endpoints of the meridians located on the cranial and facial bones of the skull.

Left: Tapping on the soft side of the hand between the wrist and little finger.

Right: Tapping on or just below the clavicle bones.

Sound Baths

Proficiency Level: ● ●
Practitioner Support:
Practitioner required
Benefits:
Blissful, Joyful, Releasing, Flowing,
Healing, Recalibrating
Equipment Required:
Singing bowls, crystal bowls,
tuning forks, gong

The fields of energy in and around the physical body can be influenced by the technology of sound as healing medicine. The physical body responds to fields of energy and when certain vibrational frequencies of sound are introduced into the field of the body, the tissues and organs will respond. Sound can be used to facilitate the movement or flow of chi in different areas of the body in order to help release physical blockages or energy stuck in the tissues.

It is understood that the vibrational frequency of injured tissues and organs, or physical or energetic blocks, is not optimal for healing or proper function. If an area of concern is surrounded by a vibrational frequency corresponding to healthy tissue, the frequency of the injury will try to entrain or synchronize with the healthy frequency being applied. The human body will automatically entrain to any external vibrational frequency, and this can affect heartbeat, circadian rhythm, breath, and other cycles of the body. This is called quantum entrainment.

Specific applications include using a gong, tuning forks, or sound bowls to tune each of the seven chakras to a specific frequency so that they become balanced and in harmony with each other. Since we are mostly composed of water, certain vibrational sound frequencies can easily penetrate the skin and be felt deep within the body. Also, the bones of the skeleton are great conductors of vibration and can transmit the applied frequencies quite readily to the arms and legs and to the skull, spine, ribs, and pelvis.

Applied Kinesiology

Proficiency Level: ● ●
Practitioner Support:
Independent/Practitioner
Benefits:
Freeing, Guiding, Calming, Confidence
Equipment Required:
None

Applied kinesiology is also known as energetic muscle testing. The energetic field surrounding the body is sensitive to anything that enters it. The effects of the external energy can either strengthen or weaken the field of the client, which in turn can affect the strength of the body itself. By noticing how the muscles of the body respond to an outside force or energy, it can be determined whether something entering the field has adverse or favorable affects.

The most common methods of muscle testing used by applied kinesiology include measuring the resistance to downward pressure by the outstretched arm, or the resistance to attempting to open the circle created by touching the tips of the thumb and forefinger. This method tends to work well for "yes" or "no" questions and for checking the compatibility of a new medicine or food with the body. Some of the effect is also due to any subconscious thoughts or feelings and may also be influenced by our intuition and gut feelings.

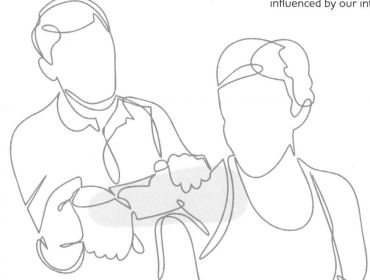

Applied kinesiology is used to test resistance in a client's body to a particular substance or their emotional response to an idea or event.

MEDITATION ENERGY THERAPIES

Meditation has become very popular because of the relaxation to be attained by being aware of the mind, body, and spirit. There are many meditation techniques, ranging from complete stillness and silence to movement and chanting.

Whether practiced laying flat or sitting up on a mat, sitting still in a chair or standing, or walking, running, or moving slowly while doing yoga or a martial art, all meditation techniques have the common goal of focusing on the breath and being present.

Right: A regular mindfulness meditation practice helps to slow your breathing and pulse, and even lower your blood pressure, leading to a reduction in stress and to a state of deep relaxation.

Mindfulness

Proficiency Level: ●
(*Beginners start here*)
Practitioner Support:
Independent/Instructor
Benefits:
Peaceful, Centering, Stillness, Relaxing
Equipment Required:
Yoga mat (optional)

Mindfulness is perhaps the least active of meditation techniques. It is usually practiced while seated, with the focus on the breath and the feelings in the body. As you begin the practice, awareness is brought to your thoughts and feelings from an observer's point of view. You may notice that as you try to quiet your mind and body, your mind might be racing or your thoughts wandering from one situation to another, worrying about the future or feeling a sense of shame or guilt about the past.

With some practice, you can begin to notice a distinction between thinking or feeling and simply being with what is so. This allows for awareness without judgment. From this state of being, the body, mind, and spirit are in harmony and your awareness becomes heightened so that you can be fully present and self-aware.

Visualization—Guided Imagery

Proficiency Level: ●
(Beginners start here)
Practitioner Support:
Independent/Instructor
Benefits:
Joyful, Blissful, Opening,
Creative, Relaxing, Healing
Equipment Required:
Yoga mat

Whether it's passive visualization or guided imagery, visualization meditation techniques can be used to create a particular state of mind that will allow you to release limiting beliefs and actually embrace the possibility of a desired future.

This technique is particularly useful for relieving anxiety around your physical health. By consciously creating a mental picture of a healthy mind and body, this may occur as if it has already happened and access to the corresponding emotional state can be achieved. The experience in and of itself can inspire and propel you into action because of the distinct possibility that it can happen.

Visualization can help to manifest a desired future by focusing on the intention and the feelings or emotions that you expect to have once your "dream" is achieved.

Psychoneuroimmunology (PNI) has shown that visualizing and imagining the white blood cells of your immune system seeking out and destroying invading infectious microbes can actually stimulate the immune response in order to combat illness and improve health. A healthy immune system is the best defense against infectious diseases.

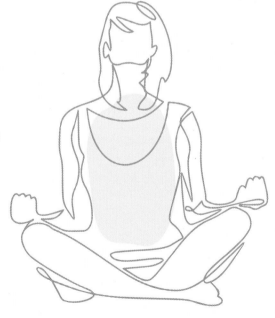

Prayer/Spirituality

Proficiency Level: ●
(Beginners start here)
Practitioner Support:
. Independent/Instructor
Benefits:
Peaceful, Joyful, Connecting,
Releasing, Gratitude, Forgiveness
Equipment Required:
Yoga mat

Prayer often has a particular goal or is a request for a specific thing or outcome. Or it could simply be to give thanks for receiving a blessing or good outcome. In either case, the goal is to achieve an active connection with a divine being greater than ourselves and to experience a level of communion that brings about feelings of gratitude, grace, and serenity.

Passive forms of silent prayer can be used to achieve a state of being that helps shut out the outside world, leading to inward contemplation and blending with an experience of exaltation as a result of a deep connection with, and even an absorption of, the divine. The repetition of a prayer can induce a state of meditation which is conducive to calming the mind and body. This in turn leads to chemical changes in the body and the resulting release of endorphins, which produces feelings of euphoria and creates an environment of healing within the body.

The experience enhances awareness of the flow of energy through the body. Physical, emotional, and energetic blocks may be released through this prayer technique.

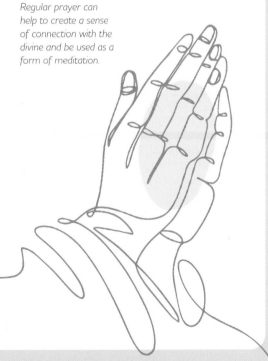

Regular prayer can help to create a sense of connection with the divine and be used as a form of meditation.

Mantra Chanting (Still Point)

Proficiency Level: ●
(Beginners start here)
Practitioner Support:
Independent/Instructor
Benefits:
Meditative, Connecting, Relaxing,
Joyful, Recalibrating
Equipment Required:
Yoga mat

Many religions around the world have used the power of mantra or sacred prayer through words to achieve a higher state of awareness, affect the subconscious mind to overcome a challenge or achieve a goal, or connect with a higher form of consciousness. This form of energy healing can help to move energy through the physical and energetic bodies.

The mantra can be spoken or sung as a prayer of invocation or a declaration. When mantras are recited as a prayer or chant, they can help reduce anxiety because you are focusing on the mantra and letting go of all other thoughts. This can be very useful as a form of meditation and can facilitate a state of deep relaxation and feelings of connectedness and wellbeing.

When the mantra is used as an affirmation, this process can help interrupt negative or disempowering thoughts or emotions by creating new thoughts that are conducive to wellbeing. Even if the mantra is a simple affirmation of being well, it can be very powerful in replacing repeating thoughts of low self-worth or overwhelm. Thoughts such as: "I'm never going to be enough," "I will never be able to accomplish my goals," "I will always be sad and unfulfilled," and "No one will ever want me" can all be replaced by "I am whole and complete," "I am in the perfect place and the universe is conspiring for my success," and "The perfect partner will show up for me at the perfect place."

Anxiety and stress can elicit the release of cortisol, which readies the body for Fight or Flight mode. This can tighten the muscles and make it difficult to relax. Energetically, reciting mantras can help remove some of the blockages or restrictions caused by anxiety and create an overall sense of wellbeing.

Mantras to try:

Om ("I am" mantra)

Om Namah Shivaya (mantra for healing)

Om mani padme hum (mantra of compassion)

Ganesh Mantra (mantra to remove obstacles):
Om Gam Ganapataye Namah

Gayatri mantra (mantra of gratitude to the sun for giving us life):

Aum Bhuh Bhuvah Svah

Tat Savitur Varenyam

Bhargo Devasya Dheemahi

Dhiyo Yo nah Prachodayat

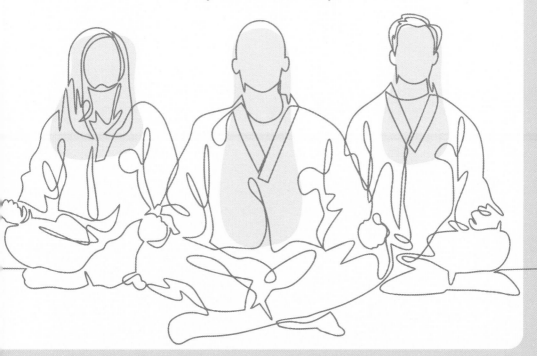

DIRECTED ENERGY THERAPIES

Non-invasive energy healing has been used throughout human history. From the healers of biblical times to modern-day shamans of the East and West, the successful stimulation of the body's healing processes through the "laying on of hands," or even through non-contact energy transfer, has been practiced with remarkable results.

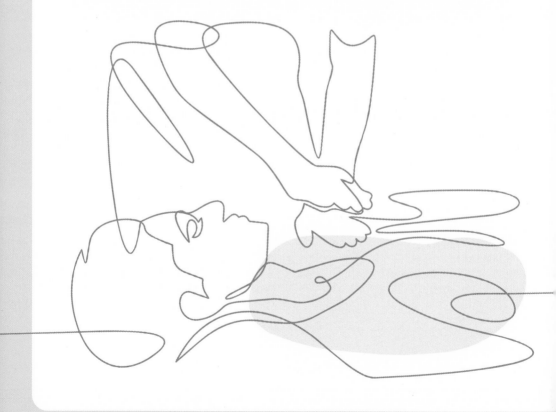

Reiki — "Universal Life Force Energy"

Proficiency Level: ● ●
Practitioner Support:
Independent/Practitioner
Benefits:
Healing, Clearing, Balancing, Protecting
Equipment Required:
None

In Reiki subtle energy therapy the practitioner may make direct contact with the client or hover inches or feet away from the body. In an even more esoteric application, the practitioner may perform the healing techniques from a long distance away without being in physical proximity to the client. This is possible because the Reiki practitioner has been "attuned" and the channels of energy transmission have been opened.

The practitioner is able to direct Universal Life Force Energy through the palms of their hands toward the site of injury or blockage. A number of mantra-like chants and symbols are used to elicit a particular response, such as boosting the Reiki energy for healing, to remove or cut ties to negative energy, to heal from a distance, or to provide emotional healing and protection.

After receiving the attunements, the practitioner heals with clear intention and invokes the Universal Life Force Energy. The client may feel surges of energy moving at a particular location in the body or a generalized flow of energy throughout the whole body.

Left: During a Reiki healing session, the practitioner will move their hands around your body. They may touch you lightly or have their hands just above your body.

Johrei—"Universal Vibration"

Proficiency Level: ● ●
Practitioner Support:
Practitioner required
Benefits:
Calming, Healing, Connecting, Flowing
Equipment Required:
None

Johrei is another non-invasive energy healing modality. This practice originated in Japan and focuses on balancing the spiritual aspects of health and wellness. The general idea is that all illness initially manifests in the energetic body and then in the physical body. If the energetic body is healed and blockages cleared, then the physical body will be healed as well.

A Johrei practitioner "sends" universal vibration energy to the "receiver." In this process, the spiritual and energetic aspects of the mind-body connection are lifted to a higher vibration and the body is able to clear blocked energies to facilitate the physical healing process. Like other subtle energy therapies, this technique acknowledges that there are fields of energy in both the "sender" and the "receiver" which both facilitate the flow of energy in the body and also encourage the innate ability of the body to heal itself.

Johrei addresses spiritual energetic issues in the energetic body which in turn influences physical health.

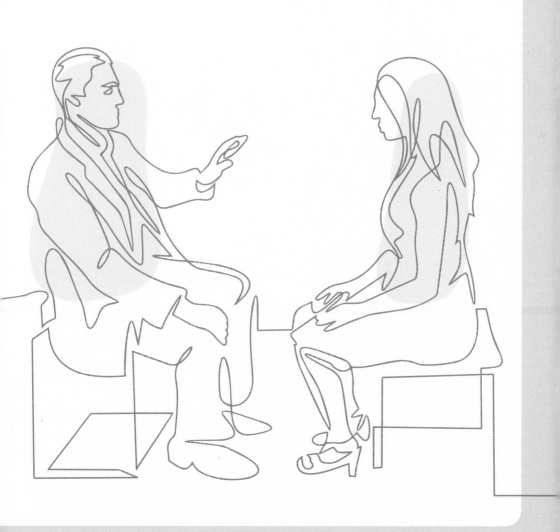

CHAPTER 4
HEALING EXERCISES

In this chapter, you will learn how to incorporate the energy healing modalities you learned about in the last chapter into your daily life. There are simple step-by-step exercises for energization, focus, pain relief, deep relaxation, and more. When performed regularly, you will notice a positive impact on your mind and body.

1

Energization Exercises

The energization exercises provide an easy and brief daily practice that incorporates 12 energetic modality components to facilitate the flow of energy to all parts of the body and promote relaxation and wellbeing.

Time 20 minutes

Level Medium

Preparation
Can be self-administered

Benefits
Energizing, balancing, relaxing, motivating

Materials/equipment None

Objective
To awaken the body, mind, and spirit. To facilitate the clearing of energetic blockages and provide focus, endurance, and increased productivity.

Useful for
Reducing stress, loosening tightness of muscles and joints. Relieving fatigue, anxiety, and depression.

Treatment method
The practice uses Earth Energy and Movement Therapies which include elements of tai chi (see page 50), qigong (see page 49), yoga (see pages 58–59), and *pranayama* breathing techniques (see page 64).

Focus
Gentle movements facilitating flow, and holding and moving energy through the toric field.
• Awareness of grounding with the Earth and connecting to the sky

with slow, deep breathing.
- Opening/softening/stretching tissues and joints.
- Balancing chakras—acknowledging the corresponding endocrine glands and five elements.

Advantages
Gentle and low impact. Can be done in a small space by all age ranges.

Drawbacks
Not recommended if wheelchair-bound.

Not good for
Back injuries, vertigo.

The Sequence

Breathe Deeply

Take five long, deep breaths, inhaling and exhaling slowly.

Focus

Awaken your relationship to the outer and inner—intention, chakras, endocrine glands

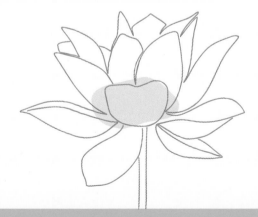

Awakening Your Energy

Stand with your feet shoulder-width apart, spine straight and long, knees soft and slightly bent (but not locked).

1 Breathe deeply.
2 Slowly raise your arms and reach upward, stretching, waving your arms from side to side, and shifting your weight from one foot to the other.
3 With arms stretched out in front of you, shake your hands and wrists, then wiggle your fingers and toes. Balance on your left foot, lift your right foot in front of you, and shake your right ankle. Press the top of your right foot into the floor, bending your toes into the ground beneath you. Switch legs and repeat.

Arm Swings

Stand with your feet shoulder-width apart, spine straight and long, knees soft and slightly bent (but not locked).

1 Breathe deeply.
2 With arms at your sides, begin to gently twist at the waist, left and then right, allowing your arms to remain limp as you twist. Gently speed up the twist for a few seconds, then gently slow down until your arms are back at your sides.
3 Lift your left arm upward and lower your right arm downward and to your side, then gently begin to swing your arms around like propellers. Start in one direction for 30 seconds and then reverse for 30 seconds. Return your arms to your sides and do the "tai-chi wave" by slowly lifting your arms in front of you as you inhale, with palms facing down, led by the wrists and with elbows bent, until they reach shoulder height. As you exhale, straighten your elbows and let your arms drop down with the palms facing forward. Repeat.
4 Place one foot in front of the other, about a foot apart, and gently begin to rock back and forth, switching your weight from one foot to the other. Let your arms remain limp as they swing forward and back along your sides for a few seconds. Switch legs and repeat.

Spine Twist

Stand with your feet slightly farther apart than your hips, lean forward slightly, and gently do a half-squat, placing your hands just above your knees and keeping a long, straight spine.

1 Breathe deeply.
2 Facing forward, draw your right shoulder down toward your left knee, allowing your left elbow to bend as you begin to look behind you, and twist to the left. Return to center and then draw your left shoulder down toward your right knee, allowing your right elbow to bend as you begin to look behind you, and twist to the right. Alternate between right and left for three cycles.
3 Breathe deeply again.

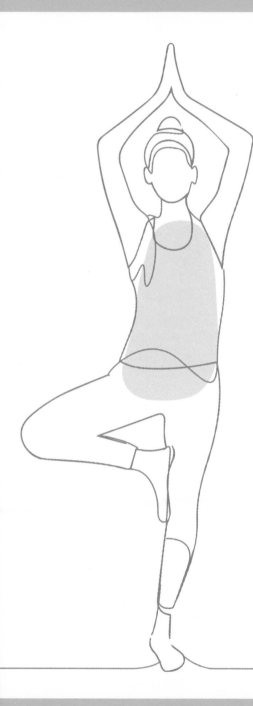

One-legged Tree

Balance on your right leg with your arms stretched upward to make a star. Bend your left knee and grab your left ankle with your right arm, then slowly lean forward as you lift your left foot behind you. Balance in this position for a few seconds, then release your ankle again and drop your arms down to your sides. Switch legs and repeat.

1 Breathe deeply.
2 Regain your balance on your right foot, bend your left knee in front of you, and grab your knee with both hands, just below your kneecap, and keep a long, straight back. Feel your hamstrings stretch for a few seconds and then release. Switch legs and repeat.
3 Breathe deeply again.

This pose give us a chance to find our center of gravity and dance around its edges.

Spine Roll-down

Stand with your feet shoulder-width apart, spine straight and long, knees soft and slightly bent (but not locked).

1 Breathe deeply.
2 Allowing your head to lead the movement, start with your knees slightly bent and slowly let your head drop, with your chin toward the sternum, engaging your quads, glutes, and abs. Bend forward, vertebra by vertebra. Feel your hamstrings stretch, and while shifting your weight from one foot to the other, allow your arms to dangle in front of you as you swing from side to side and back and forth. Swing as far forward and sideways as you can without forcing the movement, letting gravity assist you.
3 Breathe deeply again.

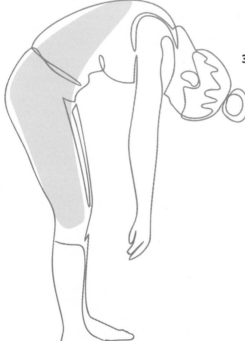

This pose stretches the back and the hamstrings, as it works the abdominals, and teaches good posture.

Spine Roll-up

Bend forward, with your feet shoulder-width apart, spine curved and long, knees soft and slightly bent (but not locked).

1 Breathe deeply.
2 Allowing your head to follow the movement, begin with your arms in a dangling position, then slowly begin to straighten your spine. Start by placing your fists behind you and pound your hips/thighs. Begin the spine roll-up, pounding first your sacrum, then your lumbar spine. Travel up your spine in this way, as high as you can reach, straightening vertebra by vertebra, chakra by chakra.
3 As you reach a standing position, pound your shoulders/neck and head, and then finish by tapping your skull and with a long, straight spine.
4 Breathe deeply again.

"1-2-3 Ha"

Stand with feet slightly less than shoulder-width apart, spine straight and long, knees soft and slightly bent (but not locked).

1 Breathe deeply.
2 With arms outstretched and palms facing down, bring your arms forward until one hand is above the other. Scissor your hands three times, inhaling with each switch. Quickly bring your arms back to an outstretched position at your sides. Rise on tiptoe as you exhale forcefully, saying, "Ha" on the fourth part of the movement. Count "1-2-3 Ha" and repeat ten times.
3 Breathe deeply again.

Finger Clasp Stretches (Front)

Stand with your feet slightly more than shoulder-width apart, spine straight and long, knees soft and slightly bent (but not locked).

1 Breathe deeply.
2 Interlace your fingers with your palms facing upward, straighten your arms, and gently pull your shoulders downward and forward. As you open up the space between your scapulas, lift your arms in front of you.
3 Switch the direction of the palms so that they are now facing downward, then straighten your arms and gently pull your shoulders downward and forward. As you open up the space between your scapulas, lift your arms in front of you.

4 Alternate between these two movements ten times. Do not FORCE the movement—allow your elbows to remain soft and bend them if need be.
5 Breathe deeply again.

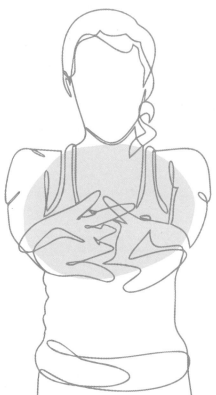

Finger clasp stretches (front and back) help to open the shoulders and facilitate a sense of release from tension.

Finger Clasp Stretches (Back)

Stand with your feet slightly more than shoulder-width apart, spine straight and long, knees soft and slightly bent (but not locked).

1   Here we will repeat the two interlaced palm movements (see Steps 1–3, page 100), this time from behind your back. Interlace your fingers with your palms facing upward, straighten your arms, and gently pull your shoulders downward and backward, pulling your scapulas together. Bend forward gently and lift your interlaced hands toward the ceiling, gently stretching the skull away from the shoulders. Do not FORCE the movement—allow your elbows to remain soft and bend them if necessary.

2   Switch the direction of the palms so that they are facing downward, then straighten your arms and gently pull your shoulders downward and backward, pulling your scapulas together. Gently bend forward and lift your interlaced hands toward the ceiling, gently stretching the skull away from the shoulders. Do not force the movement—allow your elbows to remain soft and bend them if need be.

3   Breathe deeply.

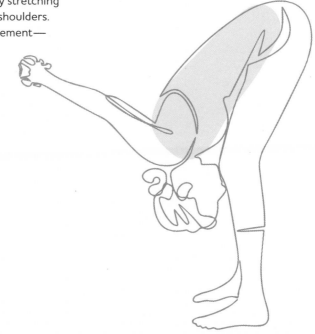

Toric Field Sweep Up (Earth)

Stand with your feet slightly more than shoulder-width apart, spine straight and long, knees soft and slightly bent (but not locked).

1 Breathe deeply.
2 With outstretched arms, lean forward slightly and gently do a half-squat, keeping a long and straight spine. Drop your arms as you reach down and gather energy with your hands from the Earth. With palms facing upward, lift the "ball of Earth energy" you have gathered in front of you up along your spine/mid-line until you reach your chest.
3 At the shoulders, twist your wrists and flip your palms downward so you can continue to push the "ball of Earth energy" up above your head and crown chakra.
4 Then slowly drop your arms down along your sides, with the palms facing downward. Repeat three times.
5 Breathe deeply again.

A chest opening, stress reducing stretch, these movements can be easily integrated into your morning routine.

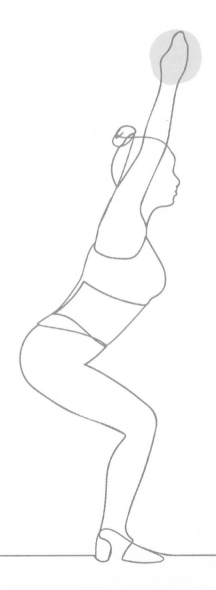

Toric Field Sweep Down (Sky)

Stand with your feet slightly more than shoulder-width apart, spine straight and long, knees soft and slightly bent (but not locked).

1 Breathe deeply.
2 Starting with your arms at your sides, reach upward along your sides with your palms facing up as you sweep your toric field upward above your head. Gather the energy from the sky and, with your palms facing downward, pull the "ball of sky energy" you have gathered down your spine/mid-line toward your chest. Continue pulling the "ball of sky energy" down toward your sacral chakra. Repeat three times.
3 Breathe deeply again.

Alternate Up/Down Toric Field Sweep

Stand with your feet slightly more than shoulder-width apart, spine straight and long, knees soft and slightly bent (but not locked).

1 Breathe deeply.
2 Start by sweeping your arms down, to gather a ball of Earth energy with your hands. Draw this essence up your spine/mid-line toward the crown chakra. Allow your arms to drop down, sweeping your toric field, then sweep your arms back up toward your crown and pull a ball of sky energy down along your spine/mid-line toward your sacrum. Repeat three times.
3 Breathe deeply again.

Conclude and kickstart your day

Close your eyes, do long deep breathing, ground and connect with your higher self, and feel your body as your temple. Be aware of your past/present/future and honor your self.

Breathe deeply.

2

Finger Qigong Exercises

Stimulate meridians and reflex points to awaken the body energetically, balance the mind, and free the spirit.

Time 5 minutes

Level Easy

Preparation
Can be self-administered

Benefits
Provides a gentle way to wake up and start your day

Materials/equipment None

Objective
To stimulate and energize the meridians and facilitate the flow of chi throughout the body and sharpen awareness and sensitivity.

Useful for
Kick-starting your energy, reducing sluggish mornings, and preparing your mind and spirit for a new day.

Treatment method
This practice uses Finger Pressure Therapies that include elements of acupressure, reflexology (see page 72), meridian stimulation, and *pranayama* breathing techniques (see page 64).

Focus
While performing the simple finger qigong exercises, imagine the flow of chi moving up and down your arms and legs. Notice the release of tension as the chi flows in the shape of the toric field through and around your body.

Advantages
Gentle and easy. Can be done
anywhere by all age ranges.

Not good for
Severe arthritis.

Drawbacks
None.

The Sequence

Finger Twist Qigong—Finger Twist and Pull

1   Grab your right index finger using
    your left hand over the top of the
    index finger. Gently squeeze and hold
    for 15–30 seconds.
2   Gently twist your index finger toward
    you. Release and repeat twice more.
3   Gently pull your index finger away
    from your wrist, holding for a count
    of three.

4   Move on to the right middle finger
    and repeat Steps 1–3 for this finger.
5   Move on to the right ring finger and
    repeat Steps 1–3 for this finger.
6   Move on to the right little finger and
    repeat Steps 1-3 for this finger.
7   Repeat the entire sequence, following
    Steps 1–6, with the left hand.

Focus

*Breathe deeply while performing the
sequence for the ultimate alignment
of body and mind*

Finger Rotation Qigong—Rotate Tips Around Each Other

1 Start with straight fingers on both hands, then spread your hands apart with only the fingertips touching.

2 Then move your wrists away from each other to make room to circle the fingertips.

3 Starting with your thumbs and using the joints at the base, part the fingertips and then circle the thumbs around each other in one direction, nine times.

4 Reconnect the tips of the thumbs and move on to your index fingers.

5 Using the joints at the base of the index fingers, circle the tips of the fingers around each other in one direction, nine times.

6 Reconnect the tips of the index fingers and move on to your middle fingers.

7 Using the joints at the base of the middle fingers, circle the tips of the middle fingers around each other in one direction, nine times.

8 Reconnect the tips of the middle fingers and move on to the ring fingers.

9 Using the joints at the base of the ring fingers, circle the tips of the ring fingers around each other in one direction, nine times.

10 Reconnect the tips of the ring fingers and move on to the little fingers.

11 Using the joints at the base of the little fingers, circle the tips of the little fingers around each other in one direction, nine times.

12 Reconnect the tips of the little fingers and move your wrists toward each other, so the base of the palms are touching. Pause for a moment to take a deep, slow breath and be present to the energy in your body.

13 Repeat the entire sequence, following Steps 1–12, but this time circle the fingertips in the opposite direction.

Finger/Toe Bending Qigong—Bend and Squeeze Fingertips

1   Grab the tip of your right thumb using the index finger and thumb of your left hand (with the left thumb on the bottom half of the right thumbnail and the pad of the left index finger on the pad of the right thumb).

2   Gently bend the tip of the right thumb toward you as you press the joint away from you, and hold for three seconds.

3   Then gently curl the joints of the thumb, moving the tip toward the palm of the hand; use the pad of the left thumb to press and hold the thumbnail down for three seconds.

4   Next, straighten the right thumb, gently squeeze the sides of the thumbnail with the left index finger and the left thumb, and, again, hold for three seconds.

5   Repeat the sequence, following Steps 1–4 for each of the four fingers of the right hand.

6   Then repeat the entire equence, following Steps 1–5 with the fingertips of the left hand.

7   Finally, repeat the entire sequence, following Steps 1–6, but this time on your toes.

When performing finger bending qigong, make sure to notice the energy between your hands. This is a subtle exercise you can do when you are in a busy environment.

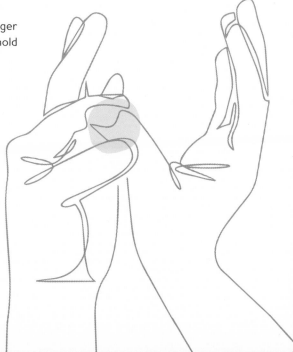

3

The Five Tibetan Rites Exercise

This is a daily routine to invigorate your chakras, awaken your joints, and supercharge your energetic flows. The Five Tibetan Rites are said to be a form of Tibetan yoga similar to the yoga series that originated in India. If you have never done this practice before, start with seven cycles. With further practice, the cycles can be increased from seven cycles to 14, and eventually from 14 cycles to 21.

Time 5–25 minutes, depending on the number of cycles

Level Medium–Difficult

Preparation
Can be self-administered

Benefits
Relieves tension, increases flexibility, opens the joints, and increases lung capacity.

Materials/equipment Yoga mat

Objective
To awaken the body using a full daily workout that will vitalize your energetic field and can be modulated for all levels of fitness.

Useful for
Opening the joints, stretching the muscles and tendons, expanding the lungs, and encouraging motility of the small and large intestines.

Treatment method The practice uses Movement Therapies that include elements of yoga (see pages 58–59), *pranayama* breathing techniques (see page 64), and chakra balancing.

Focus
The Five Tibetan Rites exercises stimulate the energetic field and awaken the organs and tissues of the body. Visualize the balanced and free-flowing movement of energy in the toric field.

Advantages

Moderate effort to strengthen your core and lower back muscles, while stretching the hamstrings and calf muscles. Works the diaphragm to facilitate deep breathing.

Drawbacks

Not recommended if wheelchair-bound.

Not good for

Requires a minimum range of motion in all joints to stay balanced.

The Sequence

RITE 1: Helicopter Spin

1 Stand with your feet less than shoulder-width apart and your arms at your sides.
2 Keeping your arms straight, lift them up from your sides, with your shoulders and palms facing downward.
3 Slowly begin spinning to your right, moving your feet to follow your spin. Try to "spot" with your head like a dancer to minimize dizziness. Spin around a total of seven times.
4 Stop spinning, then stand with your feet shoulder-width apart and place one foot slightly in front of the other.
5 Gaze at an object on the horizon in front of you and bring your hands into a "prayer-pose," with your fingers and the palms of your hands touching. Remain in this position for 30 seconds as you inhale deeply through the nose and exhale completely through the mouth.

Focus

Notice the change of energy moving through your body

RITE 2:
Head and Leg Lifts

1 Next, lie face up on a yoga mat
   with your arms at your sides, slowly
   inhaling through the nose and
   exhaling through the mouth.
2 While exhaling, slowly lift your legs
   straight up, so they are perpendicular
   to the floor, while you lift your head
   a few inches off the mat. Feel the
   contraction in your abdomen as you
   lift your legs and head.

3 Inhale as you slowly lower your legs
   and your head back to the mat.
4 Repeat Steps 2–3, as you inhale and
   exhale, a total of seven times. Then
   relax for a few moments while slowly
   inhaling and exhaling; notice the
   change of energy moving through
   your body.

*During the second
rite, it's important to
practice deep rhythmic
breathing. If you have
difficulty straightening
your knees, bend them
as needed. Try to
straighten them a little
more every time you
perform the rite.*

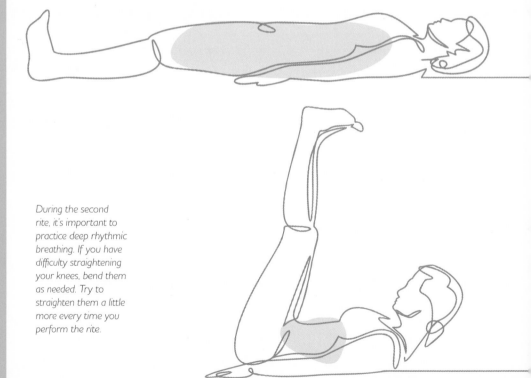

RITE 3:
Modified Camel Pose

1 Next, kneel upright on your mat, with your knees hip-width apart and your hips and shoulders in alignment with your knees.

2 Place your hands on your lower back, just above the buttocks and with your fingers pointing downward.

3 Take a moment to breathe consciously, inhaling through the nose and exhaling through the mouth, deeply and slowly.

4 While inhaling, slowly lengthen your neck and allow your head to drop backward with a slight arch in the upper back.

5 As you exhale, bring your head back into an upright position and, while lengthening your neck, allow your head to drop in front of your shoulders toward your chin.

6 Repeat Steps 4–5, as you inhale and exhale, a total of seven times.

You can also practice this rite with your eyes closed, which helps you focus inward.

RITE 4:
Modified Reverse Tabletop Pose

1   Start by sitting upright on a mat, with your legs straight in front of you, feet shoulder-width apart, and your shoulders aligned with your hips.

2   Place your hands flat on the mat, next to your hips on either side, with your fingers pointing forward toward your feet.

3   Take a moment to breathe consciously, inhaling through the nose and exhaling through the mouth, deeply and slowly.

4   While inhaling, gently lift your hips off the mat, pressing your hands and feet into the surface and bending your knees as you pull your hips toward the ceiling and allow your head to drop downward toward the mat.

5   As you exhale, allow your hips to slowly drop toward the mat and lift your head, while lengthening your neck. Allow your head to drop in front of your shoulders toward your chin, as your hips sweep the mat between your hands.

6   In one fluid motion, repeat Steps 4-5, as you inhale and exhale, a total of seven times.

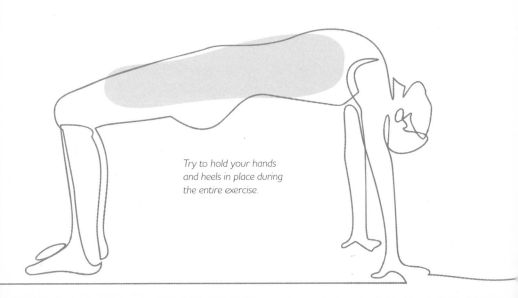

Try to hold your hands and heels in place during the entire exercise.

RITE 5:
Downward/Upward Facing Dog Pose

1   Start in a table pose, with your hands and knees on a yoga mat and both shoulder-width apart.
2   Inhale as you slowly and gently straighten your knees, keeping your arms straight and raising your hips toward the ceiling.
3   Exhale and relax the shoulders and neck, allowing a slow and gentle stretch through the backs of the legs and the small of the back.
4   Inhale as you allow your hips to drop back toward the floor while you lift your head, shoulders, and chest forward and upward toward the ceiling.
5   In one fluid motion, repeat Steps 3–4, focusing on your breath as you inhale and exhale, a total of seven times.

This rite also requires a steady breathing rhythm. To support your lower back, you can bend your knees when moving in between poses.

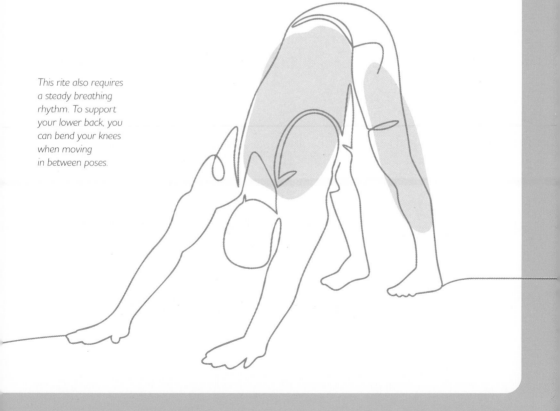

4

Deep Relaxation and Pressure Point Technique Exercises

Calm the energy of your mind, body and soul by stimulating the parasympathetic (rest/digest) response and dampening the sympathetic (fight/flight) response for deep relaxation and energetic release.

Time 25 minutes for deep relaxation, or 10 minutes for stress and anxiety reduction

Level Easy

Preparation
Can be self-administered

Benefits
Decreasing anxiety and depression

Materials/equipment Yoga mat, chair/table

Objective
To use simple and quick techniques to decrease anxiety for deep relaxation, and use acupressure points to lower blood pressure and decrease heart and respiratory rates.

Useful for
Quickly calming feelings of panic or fear and restoring balance to the mind and body.

Treatment method This practice uses Finger Pressure Therapies that include elements of reflexology (see page 72) and acupressure.

Focus
Pressure point techniques can be applied to facilitate the flow of energy and induce a state of deep relaxation and wellbeing. The mind and body will be open and relaxed and the toric field restored to a calm and peaceful state.

Advantages
Induces a calm and relaxed state that can be quickly achieved using easy finger pressure techniques.

Drawbacks
None.

Not good for
Contraindicated for low blood pressure or heart conditions.

The Exercises

Kirtan Kriya—SaTaNaMa Sequence: Spoken, Whispered, Silent, Whispered, Spoken (5 minutes each)

1 Sitting upright in a lotus pose or in a chair with your feet flat on the floor, place your hands above your knees, palms facing upward, fingers straight, and your elbows gently bent.
2 Breathing slowly and deeply, touch the tips of your thumbs with the tips of your index fingers, keeping the remaining fingers straight.
3 Then touch the thumbs with the tips of the remaining fingers in sequence, keeping the other fingers straight.
4 As you touch each fingertip with your thumb, softly repeat the mantra SAAA-TAAA-NAAA-MAAA in your speaking voice, continuing the sequence for 5 minutes.
   a. SAAA for the thumbs and index fingers,
   b. TAAA for the thumbs and middle fingers,
   c. NAAA for the thumbs and ring fingers,
   d. MAAA for the thumbs and little fingers.
5 Repeat the sequence, following Steps 4a–4d for 5 minutes, but this time, repeat the mantra SAAA-TAAA-NAAA-MAAA in a whispered voice.
6 Repeat the sequence, following Steps 4a–4d for 5 minutes, but this time, repeat the mantra SAAA-TAAA-NAAA-MAAA silently in your mind.
7 Repeat Step 5.
8 Repeat Step 4.

Reflexology: For Stress Reduction and Deep Relaxation

Shenmen point and Zero-Point
on the outer ear

1 Start in a seated position in front
of a table with your feet flat on the
floor. Center your mind and ground
yourself, connecting to the Earth
through the soles of your feet. Close
your eyes, and begin to breathe slowly
and deeply.

2 Rest your elbows on the table, then
hold the outer edge of your ears
with the index fingers and thumbs
of each hand.

3 Keeping your elbows on the table,
use the index fingers of both hands
to locate the Shenmen point in the
Triangular Valley and gently press the
Shenmen against your skull.

4 Apply light pressure to the Shenmen
(for around 2–3 minutes).

5 Release and take long, deep breaths
for 30 seconds.

6 Locate the Zero-Point in the Outer
Ridge Root and use your index fingers
to gently press the Zero-Point inward
toward your skull.

7 Apply light pressure to the Zero-Point
(for around 2–3 minutes).

8 Release and take long, deep breaths
for 30 seconds.

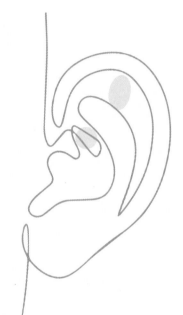

*There are more than
200 nerve ending
points in the ear,
particularly in the ear
lobes—this is why the
ear is considered a
potent reflexology zone.*

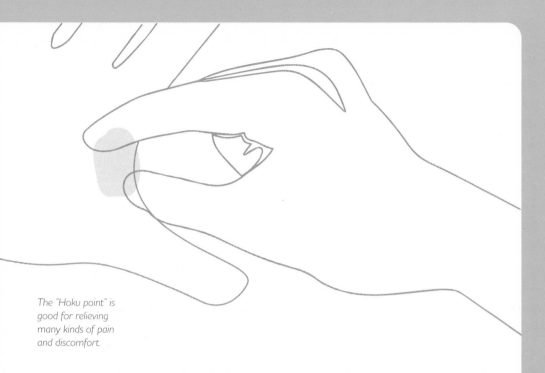

The "Hoku point" is good for relieving many kinds of pain and discomfort.

Hoku Acupressure Point on the Hand

C-clamp on the web of the hands for deep relaxation

1. Touch the tips of your left index finger and left thumb to make a circle.
2. Open the circle to form a "C" and use the tips to press the Hoku points on the web between your right thumb and your right index finger.
3. Gently press and hold the clamp for 30 seconds. You will know that you have the correct location because it will be a bit more sensitive/tender than the tissue around it.
4. Repeat Steps 1–3 using your right hand for the "C"-clamp, to gently press and hold the Hoku points on your left hand.
5. While you are holding each Hoku point, you may notice a flow of energy moving up your arm toward your chest/neck, along with a feeling of deep relaxation.

Pressure Point Techniques—Lower Blood Pressure and Stimulate PNS

Vagus Nerve Clavicle—stimulating the 10th cranial nerve

1 Sit upright with your right arm relaxed and your right hand in your lap, then begin to breathe slowly and deeply.

2 Midway along the length of your right collarbone, use your left index finger to press gently into the soft tissue just below the collarbone. Press and hold, or make small circles, with your index finger for 30 seconds.

3 Release and take long, deep breaths for 30 seconds.

4 Repeat Steps 2–3. You will know that you have the correct location because it will feel a bit more sensitive/tender than the tissue around it.

5 Repeat Steps 1–4, but this time relax your left arm instead and use your right index finger to press gently into the soft tissue just below your left collarbone.

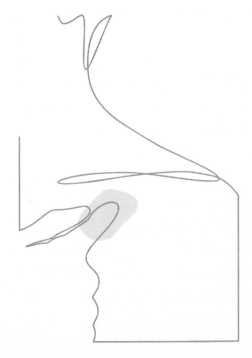

The vagus nerve sends commands to the brain and organs that slow heart and breathing rates and facilitate the motility and nutrient absorption of digestion.

Carotid Sinus Massage

1 Sit upright with your left arm relaxed and your left hand in your lap, then begin to breathe slowly and deeply.
2 Locate the carotid sinus by using the tips of your right index finger and your right middle finger to press on the right side of your neck, next to your larynx/voicebox, about half an inch to the right of the edge of your larynx. (It may help to turn your head slightly to the left and slightly upward.)
3 Gently press the tips of your fingers into the neck until you feel your pulse, then gently massage using a small circular motion for 10 seconds.

(You don't have to press hard, just enough to feel the pulse.)
4 Release and take long, deep breaths for 30 seconds.
5 Repeat Steps 2–4 one more time.
6 Repeat Steps 1–5, but this time with your right arm relaxed, using your left index and middle fingers to massage the left carotid sinus.

Try this massage to relax the pericardium (the double-walled sac containing the heart and the roots of the great vessels) and return your heartbeat to a calm and steady energetic state.

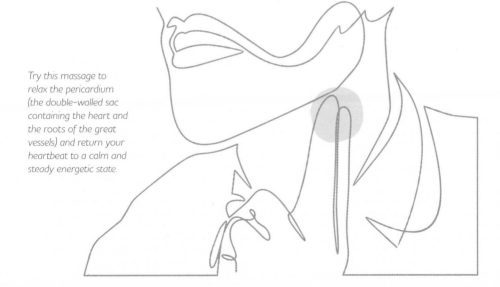

Glossary

The definitions included below are meant to provide context relative to the content in this book.

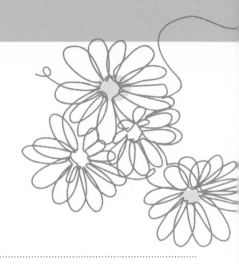

Aikido
A form of Japanese martial arts that primarily focuses on self-defense against an attacker by redirecting their energy without injuring them.

Anma
A Japanese massage practice that uses common massage techniques on the meridians and specific points of the body. Shiatsu massage originates from this practice.

Ashtanga
A series of vinyasa yoga flow exercises mainly focused on energetic ujjayi breathing, which is coordinated with the movement of the exercises.

Biofield Tuning
A sound therapy that uses tuning forks to balance the energy centers of the chakras and the nervous system as a whole. It removes energetic blockages within the body and from the energetic field surrounding the body.

Breath of Fire
A kundalini yoga breathing technique that involves short, quick inhale/exhale breathing through the nose. It is often used during kundalini yoga kriya practices.

Central Nervous System (CNS)
A body system that mainly consists of the brain and spinal cord. It integrates information being received and transmitted by all parts of the nervous system.

Chakras
Energy centers located along the spine from the cranium to the sacrum. The seven chakras correspond to neural plexuses or bundles of nerves in the body which are associated with particular organs and endocrine glands.

Chakra balancing
Performed in a range of subtle energy therapies, including Reiki, crystal healing, and sound therapy. The energy centers of the body function optimally if they are moving in harmony with each another.

Balancing the chakras helps to align the energy centers and remove any blockages.

Chi

The subtle energy that flows through the meridians of the body. It is the body's life force and is cultivated through various martial arts and *pranayama* practices.

Craniosacral therapy

A therapy that uses a gentle, hands-on approach to relieve tension in the bones of the skull and spine. It focuses on perceiving and then releasing blockages or imbalances in the dural membrane that surrounds the central nervous system.

Emotional Freedom Technique (EFT)

Also known as tapping, EFT uses percussive finger tapping on specific points of the body along with repetition of intentional phrases that correspond to an emotion related to a particular issue. The focus is on creating new neural pathways to decrease or eliminate problematic emotional or physical feelings related to the issue.

Feldenkrais Method

An exercise therapy that reorganizes or creates connections between the brain and the body. This technique can improve the efficiency and functioning of the body by using gentle, flowing movements to promote physical and psychological wellbeing.

Fight or Flight Mode

"Fight or Flight" and "Rest and Digest" are phrases used to describe responses stimulated by the sympathetic and parasympathetic nervous systems, respectively.

Jin Shin Jyutsu

A form of subtle energy work that uses gentle acupressure therapy on specific pressure points of the body to facilitate energetic flow for deep relaxation and overall health and wellbeing.

Johrei

A subtle energy healing modality that uses the hands to direct energy to "purify" the soul energy in and around the body, thus helping to heal physical illness within the body.

Jujitsu

A martial art that uses knowledge of how energy can be used both defensively and offensively against an opponent. Physical moves such as punching, kicking, and throwing are employed to leverage and direct energy as a means of subduing an opponent.

Kinesiology
The study of the biomechanical movement of the body. Kinesiology helps us understand how energy is transferred from one part of the musculoskeletal system to another. Applied kinesiology uses this understanding to muscle-test objects or ideas by stimulating the body and witnessing the energetic strength or weakness in response to the stimulus.

Kriyas
A term used by kundalini yoga practitioners to refer to a particular set of yoga exercises, including meditation, yoga poses, hand *mudras*, and mantra chants.

Kundalini
A specific yoga practice that was developed in the 1970s and which uses specific exercises (*kriyas*) to strengthen the mind, body, and soul.

Kung fu
An unarmed Chinese martial art that emphasizes both spiritual and physical elements, and utilizes self-discipline, concentration, and focus to ward off an opponent without allowing emotions or thoughts to cloud the practice.

Mantras
Sacred words or sounds that are spoken aloud and repeated for a specific number of cycles or for a specific length of time. In kundalini yoga, mantras are used as part of yoga exercises called *kriyas*.

Martial Art
Mainly East Asian in origin, a martial art consists of an ancient exercise and meditation practice of conscious body movements. These movements focus on the energetic flow of chi through the meridians and the pranic energy fields of the body.

Meridians
A network of energetic channels or vessels that run throughout the body and along which the flow of chi travels. These channels are used in Traditional Chinese Medicine, especially acupuncture, to stimulate the flow of chi, and can affect the function and health of various organs and tissues.

Mudras
Specific hand and finger positions used in a variety of meditation techniques. They are often combined with mantras for meditation.

Pilates
A relatively modern system of fitness exercises that improves flexibility, strength, and endurance. It emphasizes balancing and aligning the musculoskeletal system and strengthens the core abdominal muscles to improve posture and efficiency of movement.

Prana

The life force energy that animates all living beings. Also known as chi or "spirit energy," prana can be cultivated using *pranayama* breathing exercises to improve health and wellbeing.

Pranayama

A practice of controlled breathing techniques that can be coordinated with specific yoga movements or performed alone as a preliminary step before meditation. It sometimes includes holding the breath between the inhale and the exhale or between the exhale and the inhale for a specific length of time.

Proprioception

Also known as kinesthetic awareness, this is the ability to perceive the boundaries, movement, and position of the body in space. It is mostly unconscious and also critical to achieving the basic functions of movement.

Psychoneuroimmunology (PNI)

A multidisciplinary approach to understanding the interaction between psychological processes and their effects on the nervous and immune systems. Focuses primarily on the mental processes and their effects on the health of the body.

Qigong

A form of tai chi that uses slow, balanced, and deliberate movements of the body. It focuses on the breath and the energetic movement of chi through the body along with the flow of prana surrounding the body.

Reiki

A form of subtle energy healing that involves directing the Universal Life Force Energy toward a client to remove energetic or physical blockages in the tissues of the body, so facilitating healing and contributing to overall wellbeing.

Safety Energy Locks

A concept in Jin Shin Jyutsu that refers to 26 specific "energy sites" on each side of the body. These can be stimulated to release blockages and facilitate the flow of energy through the body.

Shiatsu

A massage technique that uses the fingers, thumbs, palms of the hands, feet, and elbows to apply pressure on specific points of the body. It includes stretching the muscles and tendons as well as the passive mechanical mobilization of the limbs to release tension, promote the healing of injuries, and decrease stress.

Sufi (yoga)

Sufism is an Islamic religion of mysticism that follows the teachings of the Koran. It includes a movement meditation that evokes a trancelike state, which results in the beautiful dance of the whirling dervishes. In this trance state, yoga (or union with the divine) can be achieved.

Tai chi

A form of martial arts that includes slow, deliberate body movements which focus on the flow of energy or chi in the body.

Taiji

A Chinese philosophy that signifies the arising of the "Supreme Ultimate" state from the "primordial universe." It seeks to reconcile and unify the elements of yin and yang energy. It balances the movement and tranquility of duality to achieve infinite potential.

Tensegrity

The state of balancing tension and compression in a system of elastic and non-elastic elements like the musculoskeletal system.

Thai yoga

A form of traditional Thai massage that incorporates therapist-assisted manipulation of the limbs and spine to mobilize the joints and also stretching to align the musculoskeletal system for the optimal and efficient motion of the body. Pressure is applied to energetic points by the therapist using their hands, legs, feet, elbows, and arms while performing the manipulation and stretching techniques.

Toric field

An energetic field generated by material objects which takes the shape of a torus. It has an axis with two poles and energy flows through the axis and around the object. The field can be affected by other fields and may have blockages and imbalances that impede the flow of energy.

Torus

A three-dimensional, geometric, ring-shaped form that closely resembles a donut.

Traditional Chinense Medicine (Tcm)

The broad and comprehensive ancient tradition of medicine in China. It focuses on the flow of chi through the meridians and involves promoting the healthy functioning of the body rather than that of the organs themselves. It incorporates forms of herbal medicine, acupuncture, martial art movement, and massage.

Ujjayi

A breathing technique that focuses on the contraction and relaxation of the diaphragm. By inhaling and exhaling slowly and deeply through the nose and narrowing the air passage in the throat, a "rushing" sound is created as air passes over the glottis.

Universal Life Force Energy

The energy of consciousness, also known as chi, ki, or prana. It is a combination of the energy of matter and the energy of spirit. It can be invoked and directed to balance and clear energy in the body and facilitate the body's ability to heal itself.

Vinyasa

A type of yoga that uses postures which focus on the flow and movement of the body. There is continuous motion during and between the postures and these are accompanied by specific breathing sequences that coordinate with the movement.

Whirling dervish

A dancer who follows the teachings of the Sufi mystic known as Rumi. Whirling dervishes spin while holding a particular posture to create an energetic field that induces a trancelike state so they can receive the blessings of the divine and impart them to observers of the dance.

Yin And Yang

In traditional Chinese philosophy these represent the duality of opposing forces which coexist as interconnected and interdependent energetic states.

Index

1-2-3 Ha exercise 99

A
absorption 66–7
acupressure 117
acupuncture 75
ailments directory 26–45
Air 62, 64
alternate up/down toric field
    sweep 103
Amyotrophic Lateral Sclerosis
    (ALS) 35
anorexia nervosa 41
anxiety 42
arm swings 96
aromatherapy 70
Attention Deficit Hyperactivity
    Disorder (ADHD) 40
autoimmune disorders 33

B
bioenergetic therapies 68–81
bipolar disease 41
blood disorders 37
blood pressure 118
body dysmorphic disorder (BDD)
    41
borderline personality disorder
    (BPD) 41
breathing techniques 64–5, 95
bulimia 41

C
camel pose, modified 111
cancer 38

cardiovascular ailments 32
carotid sinus massage 119
carpal tunnel syndrome (CTS) 44
celiac disease 33
chakras 24, 25, 120–1
chronic fatigue syndrome (CFS)
    39
Chronic Obstructive Pulmonary
    Disease (COPD) 32
connective tissue ailments 44
craniosacral therapy 76–7, 121
Crohn's disease 34
crystal medicine 69

D
dance 48, 58, 61
deep tissue massage 55
depression 42
diabetes 33, 37
directed energy therapies 88–91
downward/upward facing dog
    pose 113

E
Earth 62, 63
eating disorders 41
EFT (Emotional Freedom
    Technique) 78–9, 121
energy: awakening your 95
    definition of 14–15
    energetic flow 16–17, 62–7
    energization exercises
        94–103
    energy fields and forces 20–3
energy healing: basic principles
    of 12–25
    benefits of 11

energy meters 71
essential oils 19
exercises: deep relaxation and
    pressure point 114–19
    energization 94–103
    finger qigong 104–7
    healing 92–119
    Tibetan rites 108–13

F
Feldenkrais Method 51, 121
fibromyalgia 39
finger clasp stretches 100–1
finger qigong exercises 104–7

G
gastrointestinal ailments 34
genetic disorders 35
grounding 63

H
hands-off/on therapies 68,
    69–81
head and leg lifts 110
heart disease 32
helicopter spin 109
Hoku acupressure point 117
homeostasis 28–9

I
inflammatory disorders 33
insomnia 37
Irritable Bowel Syndrome (IBS) 34

J
Jin Shin Jyutsu 73, 121
Johrei 90–1, 121

K

kinesiology 81, 122
Kirtan Kriya 115
kundalini yoga 58−9, 122

L

leaky gut syndrome 34
lupus 33

M

mantras 86−7, 122
martial arts 48, 49−50, 122
massage 48, 54−7, 119, 123, 124
mechanical ailments 44−5
meditation: meditation energy therapies 82−7
   Sufi spinning meditation 60
   to focus direct energy healing 24−5
mental illness disorders 41
mindfulness 83
mood disorders 42
movement therapies 48−61
Multiple Sclerosis (MS) 36
Muscular Dystrophy (MD) 35

N

neurological ailments 36

O

Obsessive Compulsive Disorder (OCD) 40
one-legged tree 97

P

peripheral neuropathy 36

physiological ailments 32−9
Pilates 52−3, 122
plantar fasciitis 44
PNS, stimulating 118
polarity therapy 74
post traumatic stress disorder (PTSD) 41
prayer 85
pressure point exercises 114−19
psoriasis 33
psychological ailments 40−3

Q

qigong 48, 104−7, 123

R

reflexology 72, 116
Reiki 89, 123
relaxation exercises 114−19
restless legs syndrome 37
reverse tabletop pose, modified 112
rheumatoid arthritis 33

S

senses, energy and 18−19
shiatsu 56, 123
sight, energy and 18
skeletal alignment disorders 45
sleeping disorders 37
smell, energy and 19
social energy fields 43
sound: energy and 18−19
   sound baths 80
spine roll-up/down 98−9
spine twist 96
spirituality 85

stress, reducing 116
stroke 32
Sufi spinning meditation 60
Swedish massage 54

T

tai chi 50, 124
tapping 78−9, 121
taste, energy and 19
Thai yoga massage 57, 124
therapies: bioenergetic 68−81
   directed energy 88−91
   meditation energy 82−7
   movement 48−61
Tibetan rites exercise 108−13
toric field 20−3, 24, 25, 124
   exercises 102−3
touch, energy and 19

V

visualizations 84
   to focus direct energy healing 24−5

W

Water 62, 66−7

Y

yoga 48, 57, 58−60, 122, 124

Further Resources

Below are useful websites for additional energy medicine information and education/training.

Energy Medicine Information

Biofield Tuning
https://www.biofieldtuning.com/

Eden Energy Medicine
https://edenenergymedicine.com/

Roots and Wings Energy
https://www.rootswingsenergy.com/

The Energy Medicine Institute
https://energymedicineinstitute.org/

The Five Tibetan Rites Exercises Video
https://www.youtube.com/
watch?v=UVmhHjkHYjk&feature=emb_logo

Education/Training

Life Energy Institute
https://www.mylei.org/

The American Academy of Reflexology
http://www.americanacademyofreflexology.com/

Acknowledgments

I'd first like to thank my publishing team for their patience and giant contribution to this book. I couldn't have done it without you. I'd also like to thank my husband Steven for his amazing editorial skills, which helped me find my voice and say what I mean in a way that others actually understand.

I am also grateful to one of my many teachers who taught me to remember to "trust and allow." This alone gets me through many challenges, great and small.

And, finally, it is with deep gratitude that I honor the guidance and clarity provided by the unseen Universal Life Force Energy, which allows me to continue being of service and to offer the gift of energy healing to all.

Illustration credits: